SELF-TRACKING

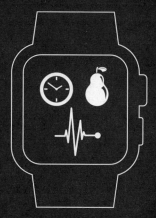

The MIT Press Essential Knowledge Series

SELF-TRACKING

GINA NEFF AND DAWN NAFUS

The MIT Press | Cambridge, Massachusetts | London, England

This book was set in Chaparral Pro by the MIT Press. Printed and bound in the United States of America.

Library of Congress Cataloging-in-Publication Data

Names: Neff, Gina, 1971– author.
Title: Self-tracking / Neff, Gina, and Dawn Nafus.
Description: Cambridge, MA : MIT Press, 2016. | Series: The MIT Press essential knowledge series | Includes bibliographical references and index.
Identifiers: LCCN 2015039937 | ISBN 9780262529129 (pbk. : alk. paper)
Subjects: LCSH: Patient self-monitoring. | Self-monitoring. | Self-care, Health—Technological innovations. | Medical telematics. | Medical innovations—Social aspects. | Information technology—Social aspects.
Classification: LCC RA418.5.M4 N44 2016 | DDC 610.285—dc23 LC record available at http://lccn.loc.gov/2015039937

10 9 8 7 6 5 4 3 2 1

CONTENTS

SERIES FOREWORD

The MIT Press Essential Knowledge series offers accessible, concise, beautifully produced pocket-size books on topics of current interest. Written by leading thinkers, the books in this series deliver expert overviews of subjects that range from the cultural and the historical to the scientific and the technical.

In today's era of instant information gratification, we have ready access to opinions, rationalizations, and superficial descriptions. Much harder to come by is the foundational knowledge that informs a principled understanding of the world. Essential Knowledge books fill that need. Synthesizing specialized subject matter for nonspecialists and engaging critical topics through fundamentals, each of these compact volumes offers readers a point of access to complex ideas.

Bruce Tidor
Professor of Biological Engineering and Computer Science
Massachusetts Institute of Technology

ACKNOWLEDGMENTS

One of the key points of this book is that knowledge—even about the self—is a social product. So, too, of course, is this little book, which was made possible only through the contributions and efforts of many. While this book is a primer and not a work of ethnography, many people have been extraordinarily generous with their time, teaching us their perspective, sharing their views on data, and helping us understand what the stakes are. The dedication of patient advocates, data activists, and quantified-self enthusiasts inspires us with a view of what is possible when people get involved in the technologies that matter to them.

Margy Avery first encouraged us to think about how to communicate the issues of self-tracking for the general reader. Without her keen editorial instincts we would have never taken on this project. Susan Buckley and Gita Manaktala helped shape and guide it from sketchy proposal to the finished product. Kathleen Caruso once again proved to be an extraordinary manuscript editor seemingly capable of managing every possible contingency with grace and attention to detail, and the keen eye of copyeditor Julia Collins improved this book tremendously. Shannon O'Neill and Will Lippincott at Lippincott Massie McQuilkin worked with us to clarify our ideas for the general audience and ensured that they made it into print. For that we are both exceedingly grateful.

We thank Brittany Fiore-Gartland, Kristen Barta, Chris Monson, and Peter Nagy for contributing vital research assistance for projects related to this work and for marshaling the gush of news media on the quantified self. This work has also benefited greatly from the generosity of anonymous peer reviewers whose investments of time and thought into our ideas strengthened this book and its argument.

Dawn would like to thank the many self-trackers whose experimentation has taught us so much. In particular, Anne Wright has been extremely clear, thoughtful, and helpful in showing what it takes to do self-tracking in ways that solve an actual problem. Rajiv Mehta has been inspiring to work with over the years. Steven Jonas expanded our imagination about the ways that self-reflection could happen through data, and the folks at QS Labs have provided incredibly stimulating, thoughtful, and usefully challenging conversations. Dawn would also like to thank her colleagues at Intel, and particularly the Data Sense team—Sangita Sharma, Lama Nachman, Pete Denman, Rita Wouhaybi, Lenitra Durham, Evan Savage, Devon Strawn, and Tim Coppernoll. John Sherry contributed to this work as both lab leader and valued mentor. Jamie Sherman, Yuliya Grinberg, Dana Greenfield, Minna Ruckenstein, and Whitney Erin Boesel have shaped much of the thinking presented here. Jim and Penni Nafus provided the much deeper foundation on which this work has been based. Dan

Jaffee deserves special thanks for his support during the troubling time through which this book was written. To the good friend who had the unfortunate task of having to point out what was right there and yet somehow so very difficult to see, Dawn extends her gratitude for this person's honesty and collaboration.

Gina would like to thank numerous colleagues who have helped clarify the ideas presented here, including discussions after talks at Princeton and Stanford. Colleagues at the School of Public Policy at Central European University and the incredible students there pushed the public implications of the quantified self to the fore. Her research on self-tracking and personal data was supported by Intel, the Center for Information Technology Policy at Princeton University, and the Institute for Advanced Study at Central European University. The University of Washington Rome Center and the Raul Wallenberg Guesthouse in Budapest provided space to write the first draft of this book, and particular thanks go to Éva Gönczi, Éva Fodor, and Ágnes Forgó. Phil Howard and our sons Hammer and Gordon make time spent writing possible, enjoyable, and worth the effort.

Finally, we both would like to thank readers for picking up this book, and we urge them to get involved in the issues at hand.

AN INTRODUCTION
TO SELF-TRACKING

People now keep track. An array of numbers follows us through each day. Hours slept. Steps walked. Hours billed and minutes concentrated. People friended. Tweets sent. There is a veritable explosion of self-directed tracking. A whopping 110 million wearable sensors will be shipped by the end of 2016.[1] Weekend athletes now race each other virtually, while office workers keep track of how much of their computer time is spent goofing off on social media and how many followers their posts reach. Homeowners keep track of how much energy each appliance uses, while glucose monitoring is no longer done just by diabetics. Why do so many people do these things?

This book examines self-tracking—how and why people record, analyze, and reflect on data about themselves. We share some of the emerging research on this area of social life, looking at what people actually do with data about themselves, the tools they use, and the communities they become part of in the process. We show how data can be useful, powerful, tedious, pleasurable, underwhelming, wrong, or just beside the point in a variety of everyday contexts. We also explore what happens when data gets caught up in institutional relationships. Firms, universities, governments, and other types of organizations are all involved in producing or handling data. We focus on self-tracking primarily as it relates to wellness and health, for that is the sort of data that people tend to care most deeply about, and where the debates about the social implications are the most intense. We aim to explain why there is so much enthusiasm for the power of data in people's hands, and consider critics' important cautions about how it can also go very wrong.

Self-tracking is a human activity, one far more interesting than the gadgets that have made it easier and more widespread. Self-tracking does not necessarily require technology more complex than pen and paper. However, much self-tracking is now digital, whether done via wearable computers, like smartwatches and fitness bands, or mobile phones or computers. These technologies intersect with the ways that people have self-tracked for centuries like keeping diaries or logs. The growth of these digital traces raises new questions about this old practice. The technologies extend the areas of life that can be measured, and they make it possible to keep track with greater frequency than ever before. It is only when we look at how the practices and the tools come together that we can see how a new social phenomenon emerges.

Self-tracking takes place in social situations. The numbers of self-tracking may focus on the individual, but they stem from fundamental beliefs about how societies function. The relationships between technology users and manufacturers inform what kinds of technologies eventually become available. The relationships between doctors and patients inform how the data that people keep about their bodies is used in clinics. People in the roles of technology users, producers, patients, and medical professionals each have their own social circles or communities that they consult to make sense of what self-tracking is "really" about. In these communities, self-tracking tools are being built, and the practices are being shaped. For that reason, we spend time looking at some of the social dynamics there.

Why We Wrote This Book

We met on a clear January morning in San Francisco to write together. As we walked to breakfast, Gina (a sociologist of technology and communication scholar working in academia) talked of the odd experience of walking into a Best Buy store in Lexington, Kentucky, just before Christmas and seeing what has become a staggering array of the objects we study: activity trackers, heart sensors, sleep monitors, bike monitors, baby monitors. What were, ten years ago, glimmers of ambition in otherwise awkward prototypes have now become the latest new thing to buy for someone as a gift. (See the photographic evidence of such displays in figure 1.1.) Dawn (an anthropologist, working in industry to inform technology development) mentioned that her local weekly newspaper, the *Portland Mercury*, had a cover story on "health goths," a perplexing mix of youth "emo" subculture, dourness, and, apparently, Nike Fuelbands. Goths are self-tracking? How on earth did that happen? As we struggled to imagine the incongruity of striving, athletic, all-black-clad goths, Dawn tripped, falling to the ground. When she tried to rise, we realized something was not right. Really, really not right. There, directly in front of the fancy San Francisco coffee shop that had been our destination, we waited for an ambulance while off-duty techies within waited for their siphon-bar brewed coffees and quinoa breakfast salads.

The thing about a broken kneecap is that it requires painkillers—a mix of them. It's a complicated cocktail of different pills on different cycles, with varying risks to the liver, breathing, and gut. A few hours after the first pill, Dawn takes another. Then a few hours later, she wonders: Is it safe to take the next pill? She can't remember two pills back. And what of the daily allotment of the liver-damager? It doesn't matter when you take that one, but it

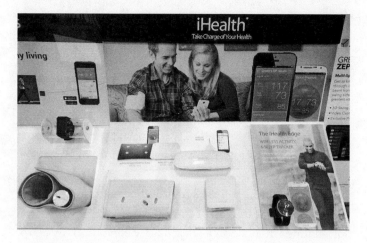

Figure 1.1 Christmas display of self-tracking tools, Best Buy, Lexington, Kentucky.
Source: Gina Neff.

does matter how many you take per day. There is no keeping track in the head, and the pills themselves discourage clear-headedness. Having studied self-tracking for years, Dawn's instinct for how to solve this problem is to do some manual tracking—that is, writing things down without using a sensor to keep track automatically. She has an app on her phone where she can enter a number or some text, which is stored alongside a time stamp. She decides to enter the name of each medicine. When she views the record, she's able to count backward the hours since she took that kind of pill, keeping all the different cadences running, but not in her head. For the liver-damager, she's less concerned about the hours since the last pill, and more concerned about keeping the total pills she consumes for the day under the recommended number. So for those she counts how many, not how long since. Some weeks later, she shows all this to a curious visitor. "Huh," he says. "I see why you did that, but I gotta say, I probably wouldn't have thought to do that myself." Dawn doesn't think she would have either, if she hadn't been writing this book.

In 2014, Gartner, a technology industry research group, put wearables at the top of their "Hype Cycle," a widely followed index of Silicon Valley industry bloviation. By 2015, they had entered Gartner's "trough of disillusionment," a phase full of doubt that they say precedes long-term adoption of a technology. Meanwhile, social scientists and philosophers joined in studying how wearables are being sold and used, and began to point out their problems. They were particularly concerned about how scientific transparency was being glorified at the expense of other values, creating an illusionary reduction of human life to numbers. They began to worry that individuals were being asked to bear the burden of managing risks they had very little practical control over—a social dynamic they had seen in many, many other spheres of life. They raised concerns about the tremendous power given to already powerful corporations when people allow companies to peer into their lives through data. Self-tracking, social scientists and critics worried, gives far too much power to those who decide what is worth measuring and who measures up. Yet when Dawn's disaster struck, the ability to self-track was no longer just a topic of academic conversation or industry hype. It was something that *mattered*, in a very practical and personal way. This ability was more than an object purchased off the shelves of a major retailer, but it was also that, too.

Journalist Nora Young was perhaps the first to notice this key tension in self-quantification.[2] Digital traces of our every move can lay the groundwork for terrible social consequences, such as rampant privacy violations, the commodification of daily living, "healthism" (the fetishization of anything and everything deemed healthy),[3] and a preoccupation with the personal that erodes our capacity for coordinated community action. But Young also noted that there is much about self-quantification that is actually useful for both individuals and communities. Keeping track of medicines spared Dawn's liver, and later we will see how coordinated data efforts sometimes lead to better medical knowledge and, occasionally, more equitable participation in medical practice.

We grew concerned about this tension both as people who use data in our own lives, and as social scientists who have examined the social entanglements people get involved in when they make and use data. We felt that this tension between usefulness and social complications created a need for an introductory book on the topic that gathered together the existing research, the relevant journalism, and other materials. Wider public participation in the debates that surround self-tracking could tip the balance toward things working in the public interest. The choices we make in our day-to-day lives about what data to collect matter for what other people can do with that data, and how it might be used against us. When we do not actually have a choice about what data is collected, or about where our data goes, our ability to raise our voices as citizens begins to matter even more.

The public interest in self-tracking could be thought about as something broad and civic-minded like privacy policy, or a concern about surveillance. However, it also has to do with social relationships much closer to home. Self-tracking data refers to an individual person, but it is fundamentally social. Consider just how many people are affected if an individual uses one of the many sensors now available to determine indoor air quality. A home device monitoring air quality captures data on substances present in interior spaces, including potentially harmful ones like carbon monoxide or even toxins from industries located in other regions, possibly even other countries. Indoor air quality affects the health of everyone in the house, and potentially visitors, too. Each person might be affected differently by the particular substances tracked by the device, and having data might change how people in that house talk about their health with one another. But changing air quality might not be something that an individual home-owner can tackle alone. A problem might ultimately need to be solved through local, national, or even potentially international efforts—and who pays for this is likely to be controversial.

Air quality is not the only type of data that implicates others. Most data does. Even genetics data reflects and reveals things about our immediate and extended families, and individuals who choose to get their genome analyzed effectively choose for their families as well. Many times self-tracking is talked about as an individual (sometimes narcissistic) pursuit, but the data generated has implications for many other people. At stake here are the very lenses we use to see ourselves and others. The ability to design or use those lenses with care can make or break important relationships.

There are also many unknowns to contend with, some to do with the nature of the emerging technology, and others to do with how uncertain data is handled societally. Sometimes our capacity to gather data outpaces our ability to make sense of it. Data collection on the genome, microbiome (the bacteria in the gut thought to influence everything from obesity to mental health), and exposome (the pollutants that bodies are exposed to) has outpaced science's understanding of their effects on the body. How will people handle such uncertainties? What will they demand of their doctors and healthcare systems? How will

At stake are the very lenses we use to see ourselves and others.

they challenge scientists and experts, or mobilize scientific expertise? What governmental and social responses will they expect?

While the unknowns are debated, there will be many situations in which people look to self-tracking to fit their specific needs. Mothers will watch their babies grow, in the flesh but also through numbers. Athletes will seek to up their "game." People with diabetes will simply want to get through their days safely. In each case, tracking is different and different goals must be met. Tracking requires a system of some kind—a mobile phone, pen and paper, sensors, memory. Some people may buy a device or download an app looking to solve a problem, identify a glitch, or encourage a habit. The problem as we see it is that many off-the-shelf tracking options, sold through appeals to "empowerment," do not actually help people figure out which questions they should be asking, much less how to ask the next question, test ideas, or make discoveries. As a result, few people are getting out of their self-tracking devices what they hoped they would, but they are also incurring some of the societal costs and burdens that the social scientists are starting to point out.

This situation is not a necessary or final state of affairs. We hope to offer information about the essential ideas and challenges of self-tracking to support wider participation in the debates. We do this in two ways. The first is to show, based on our research and that of others, what people do when they manage to meet their own needs successfully with self-tracking. This doesn't require special technical skills or scientific knowledge, but there is a set of approaches that can work well for many people, and we share them here. The second is to point out those areas within communities of medical practice, commercial activity, and policy making where more public involvement could potentially effect change so that self-tracking tools further, rather than undermine, the public interest.

Each of the authors has different expertise that grounds our introduction of self-tracking. The research we draw on in this book, including our own, is cultural and social—not behaviorist or strictly technological. In our fields we try to understand how people make sense of the situations they find themselves in, and how they come to the beliefs that they hold. The research we draw on here tends to observe and talk with people in their "natural" settings, as opposed to lab experiments.

In terms of our individual backgrounds, Dawn ran a research team that investigated consumer adoption of a new kind of technology called biosensors, which have numerous self-tracking applications. Like many anthropologists who work outside universities, she applies ethnography to design and business questions. She now co-leads a combined engineering and ethnographic research project to understand how design might better support new forms of data. She also has been an active participant in the

Quantified Self (QS) community, a group for people who self-track. The firm she works for, Intel, has been a sponsor of QS and makes technical components for self-tracking technologies. Mixing intellectual commitments with commitments to a community and with a day job is, as we show in chapter 4, not unusual in self-tracking. While this applied work deepens a person's knowledge about the design choices available, it also creates a point of view that has its own limitations. Gina is a sociologist of communication technology working for a university. Gina worked with Dawn on the biosensors project, focusing primarily on the field site of digital health innovation. She looked at how self-tracking is blurring the line between home and clinic and how regulation affects the relationship between medical practice and self-care. She focuses on the analysis of industries and social institutions on how technology is used in practice.

As with any introductory text, this book is informed by the inclinations and preoccupations of its authors. It is highly probable that we left out important topics or areas of debate, either because we are ourselves unaware of them, because the literature was too nascent to have much to say about it, or because the works emerged after we wrote this book. It is also likely that we emphasized some matters more than others because our respective disciplines are more attuned to those matters, or because of the roles we play in the communities we are in, or because we ourselves are just as influenced by social conditions as the other people we talk about in these pages. No researcher, no matter how careful, can avoid these factors influencing what she chooses to research, and the approaches that seem reasonable.

We think that sociological and anthropological perspectives are helpful if we want to understand why, for example, people abandon their activity trackers after a few months or leave fitness apps closed on their smartphones. The market successes and failures of self-tracking tools are neither coincidences nor so-called user failures. While plenty of techniques use insights from psychology to increase individual users' engagement with those products, there is also a set of social arrangements that explain why, even after these techniques are used, so many people put self-tracking tools in a drawer after a few weeks' time. These very same social patterns, or cultural habits of thought, also inform debates about data ownership, access, privacy, and the rightful place of medicine and commerce in society. Such debates determine whether data can be used against the very people whose bodies generated it. They also determine who can and cannot participate in medical research and breakthroughs, who gets to decide what is learned from data, and who challenges scientific authority. To move the public debates forward, it helps to understand not just what the participants are saying, but also what they are assuming about how people, technologies, communities, and societies work. This is the contribution the social sciences can make, and what we hope to introduce with this book.

We Have Always Been Quantified

Quantifying is not new. Benjamin Franklin, the eighteenth-century US statesman, kept accounts of how he spent his time and whether he lived up to the virtues he set forth for himself. His tracking, in charts and short notes, was "the execution of this plan for self-examination."[4] Such daily tracking in the form of diaries was common, and in fact, eighteenth-century diaries were written to be shared and were made up of relatively brief entries, personal logs with short facts laid out sequentially. Communication scholar Lee Humphreys and her coauthors found that today's Twitter feeds bear a great resemblance to eighteenth- and nineteenth-century diaries in how both "account, reflect, communicate and share with others using media of the times."[5] Although his style was very different from Benjamin Franklin's, the mid-twentieth-century inventor Buckminster Fuller also quantified himself by creating a giant scrapbook of sorts, rigorously archiving something or other once every fifteen minutes. In a sense, these two styles exemplify different threads of self-tracking that continue today, one where the data plays an active role in changing one's life and the other where it plays a more passive role to support personal reflection. Today we might call Franklin's approach "self-tracking" and Fuller's approach "life-logging," a close cousin to self-tracking that can, in fact be more interventionist than we might at first suppose. Franklin's approach to what we would now call self-tracking had noninstrumental and contemplative aspects that look more like "life-logging" than it might at first seem. To these two histories we must add a third—that of active self-experimentation. Before the modern clinical trials were conducted on thousands of people, self-experimentation was a major part of scientific work. Sir Isaac Newton nearly blinded himself staring into a reflection of the sun to try to understand the workings of the eye. Ibuprofen, malaria vaccines, and neuroscience all have self-experimentation as part of their contemporary histories, and important discoveries continue to be made by self-experimentalists. All three of these—self-tracking, life-logging, and self-experimentation—influence how we view knowledge about the self, and each has a history.

This element of experimentation has always raised debates about who has knowledge, and what is valid knowledge. Data in more people's hands is not neutral; it can create or undermine beliefs. Proponents of contemporary self-experimentation argue that self-experimentation is not a lesser form of science. It can be done in settings more realistic than lab-based experiments, and facilitate more longitudinal work. Skeptics, however, believe that self-experimentation insufficiently removes bias, as the experimenter is both research subject and interpreter of the research data. Accusations of bias should always be taken with a grain of salt, however. Scientific paradigms shift not just through more evidence (evidence that may have been there all along if scientists looked at it in a certain way), but also through changes in beliefs. Historical examples can remind us of just how difficult it is to untangle belief in the evidence from belief in the people offering said evidence. In medieval England, for example, female healers discovered that putting bread on wounds assisted healing (penicillin, anyone?). Their gender meant they were accused of witchcraft, not scientific discovery, but in this case they were well ahead of "proper" scientists who were still working with the four humors of Hippocratic medicine. Similarly, when indigenous groups around the world develop ethnobotanical knowledge, these practices are sometimes remarkably biologically effective, and sometimes not. Scientists who work with these plants sometimes rely on the existing indigenous knowledge about them, and sometimes dismiss that knowledge out of hand.

In some of the examples we will read about, people use self-tracking practices to discover something that helps them in ways that Western science does not. In other cases, what they do corroborates, or relies on, what is already known. Societal biases continue to be revealed in the places where people give the benefit of the doubt in cases they shouldn't, or ignore discoveries because they come from unsavory or unlikely sources. Belief and evidence to the contrary can sit side by side, noticed or unnoticed, in both scientific and lay circles. A further goal of this book is to show how self-experimentation with data forces us to wrestle with the uncertain line between evidence and belief, and how we come to decisions about what is and is not legitimate knowledge.

If quantification has always been with us, what is new about self-tracking? The first new development is a change in technology. The ability to electronically sense a wide variety of phenomena has been an ongoing goal of engineering and computer science. The advent of the mobile phone as a computational platform, miniaturization of sensors and the other components of sensor systems, and improvements in connectivity infrastructure and data storage have all created the conditions that make the widespread use of sensors conceivable. The interdependencies are so intricate that it truly is astounding that we have working sensor systems at all, let alone an extensive market for them.

The second development is a cultural change, *biomedicalization*, which is the extension of medical or biological explanations for the way things are.[6] It is now hard to find corners of life that are not subject to biomedical interpretation, from moods and feelings to life success itself. Biomedicalization has taken over as a mental model, a habit of thought that makes medicine the most readily available explanation for why things are the way they are. In a biomedicalized world, it is easier to acknowledge the impact of a cluster of neurons than the impact of culture or society on why people behave in the way that they do. This extensive process of biomedicalization carves a groove in our collective imagination that makes close measurement of the body both conceivable and desirable. "Health," in turn, has become a loaded word, not merely a description of a bodily state but also a euphemism for what the speaker believes is or is not desirable. Being told your "behavior is not healthy" can be incredibly shaming—you have just been told you have broken the social rules of a biomedicalized world. Biomedicalization is also an intensely powerful social force that has influenced the technology market. Even though only a small portion of self-tracking tools is used for medicine, most of these tools draw on biomedicalized understandings and frameworks. In this way, biomedicalization has found its way onto the consumer electronics shelf.

Communities and tools inform what people can and cannot do when they self-track. There might be technical limitations on what is possible to track, or being situated in a community can make some things appear more important to track rather than others. Next we will present some

Biomedicalization carves a groove in our collective imagination that makes close measurement of the body both conceivable and desirable.

of the basic outlines about what people do when they self-track, the tools that they use, and the communities that shape self-tracking. These outlines help set the stage for chapter 2, which delves into some of the broader societal issues that self-tracking tools raise.

The Practices

What people actually do with their data is an important question for two main reasons. First, ordinary people discover and learn things by trying stuff out, just as much as engineers and researchers do. What they learn informs our shared understandings of what data means. Second, what people do with data matters as a kind of economic activity. A market does not just exist "out there" without people—there is communication between sellers and buyers, where ideas and skills concerning how to use these things are exchanged. This market is a place where long-standing ideas about the body, about science, and about visual forms are all put into practice, and changed as a result.[7]

Keeping track often involves using new gadgets, but it is interesting to note that the people who are most inclined to use new gadgets—called "lead users" in some circles—tend to be interested in tracking the same things as the broader public. A nationally representative survey and an analysis of videos from the Quantified Self community

Table 1.1

Examples of self-tracking projects and motivations from QS

Motivation	Subcategories	Tracking example
Improve health	Cure or manage a condition	Track blood glucose to hit the target range
	Achieve a goal	Track weight to get back to the ideal weight
	Find triggers	Log triggers that cause arterial fibrillation
	Answer a specific question	Track niacin intake dosage and sleep to identify how much niacin to take for treating symptoms
	Identify relationships	Track exercise, weight, muscle mass, and body fat to see the relationship
	Find balance	Log sleep, exercise, and time to get back from erratic lifestyle
Improve other aspects of life	Maximize work performance	Track time to know the current use of time/find ways to be more efficient
	Be mindful	Take a self-portrait shot every day to capture each day's state of mind
Find new life experiences	Satisfy curiosity and have fun	Log the frequency of puns to see what triggered them
	Explore new things	Track every street walked to explore the city
	Learn something interesting	Track heart rate as long as possible to see what can be learned

Source: Eun Kyoung Choe, Nicole B. Lee, Bongshin Lee, Wanda Pratt, and Julie A. Kientz, "Understanding Quantified-Selfers' Practices in Collecting and Exploring Personal Data," in *Proceedings of the 32nd Annual ACM Conference on Human Factors in Computing Systems* (Toronto, Canada: ACM, 2014), 1143–1152.

of self-trackers show striking similarities between the self-identified "self-trackers" and the wider population in terms of what and why people track. Both studies found people predominantly tracked physical activity, food, and weight.[8] In table 1.1 we summarize the findings on what people said that they were trying to accomplish with self-tracking, which ranged from improving their health or their life to finding new life experiences.

While there is a good deal of diversity in self-tracking, there is a a common "lifecycle" of data, in which people collect, synthesize, analyze, and reflect on data.[9] Similarly, a Carnegie Mellon University team identified key challenges that lead users of self-tracking faced. These include collecting the data they wanted (e.g., when to enter data, fiddling with device charging), integrating the data so they could make sense of it (e.g., how do you even get it all in one place?), and looking at the data (e.g., setting aside time to reflect, not liking what they saw).[10] Casual self-trackers might be even less determined to get what they need from tracking devices. According to a PricewaterhouseCoopers (PwC) survey, 21 percent of the US population uses some type of wearable, but only 10 percent actually use the wearable daily.[11] In 2012, 60 percent of health-related apps fell into disuse after six months.[12] The technology industry has been aware of widespread early abandonment for a number of years now.[13] Academic research also identifies how self-tracking tools fail to "engage" their users. We discuss why the technology industry struggles to increase user engagement in chapter 4.

Still, there are triumphant industry and media reports that indicate strong demand for technologies that support health and wellness (again, ignoring all the other things that self-tracking can actually do). Roughly half of surveyed Americans claimed to believe that wearable technology could improve life expectancy by ten years (56 percent), assist in reducing obesity (46 percent), or increase athletic capacity (42 percent).[14] Clearly, then, the industry's messaging that data products solve health problems is getting through, even if these problems are not being solved in practice. The assumption that tracking leads to the ability to see a deficiency, and that in turn leads to the ability to act, dominates business models and technology design for self-tracking. However, the rate that people abandon tracking suggests they also do not believe this model is adequate when it comes to their own bodies. The fantasies of being able to reduce obesity or increase longevity solely with the introduction of technology are beginning to confront the realities of how people use these tools in practice.

Some researchers argue that what people are "really doing" when they self-track is demonstrating to themselves that they can properly manage their own affairs and can control their body in socially acceptable ways.[15] Others describe self-tracking as a practice of outsourcing the task of bodily management to technologies, where people relieve themselves of the burden of thinking about it.[16] Still others would like to see technologies limit themselves to serving as "prosthetics of feeling," focused on in-the-moment mindfulness as opposed to an intellectually driven quest for insight.[17] Our own stance is that data should be thought of as a kind of transducer.[18] An electronic transducer makes a digital reading by preserving some qualities of an electrical signal, but only some. Smoke is not the same thing as fire, but sometimes it does in fact indicate fire. Similarly, in data some things get communicated while others get lost. There is much room for people to maneuver in the imperfect translation.

An important aspect of what people do with self-tracking is how others inform what they do and why they do it. Sometimes self-tracking is not an individual action even though the name might imply that. There is a wide range of situations where the "self" in self-tracking is driven out by other interests and power dynamics, and the practice starts to become "other-tracking." Sociologist Deborah Lupton identifies a continuum between fully self-driven and abject commercial exploitation, usefully identifying what could lie in the middle.[19] *Communal tracking* or what increasingly is referred to as "citizen science" involves donating privately tracked data to public health research for the greater good. Open Paths, for example, is a project that helps users secure their own data from multiple mobile and digital sources and then choose which research project, if any, to donate their data to. *Pushed tracking* can be where people are given economic incentives—such as when employers "incentivize" employees through various sticks and carrots to self-track—or receive social pressure that makes the cost of not tracking high. Children are sometimes asked to self-track by their parents, or their parents keep track on their behalf, either for medical or other reasons. There may indeed be valid reasons for parents to do this, but children have less ability than adults do to give meaningful consent. *Imposed tracking* is when there is no meaningful alternative, such as when activity tracking becomes a prerequisite for employment or insurance coverage.

Where the concerns of self-trackers and the others who have access to their data are not well aligned, these become matters for a more vigorous public policy discussion. This is where the more serious negative social consequences can happen, and where we might see practices involving more active resistance. Recent experiences with body cameras used by police, dash cams on police cars, and bystanders' mobile phone cameras indicate that it is possible for the tools of surveillance to be turned around and used for *sousveillance*, or watching the powerful from below. Who watches whom is not yet settled.

The Tools

By tools, we mean any device that can be used for collecting, analyzing, and making sense of self-tracking data from pen and paper to a "lab on a chip," where new developments in microfluidics make it possible to test blood, saliva, or other fluid without sending samples off to labs. There have been many important changes in self-tracking technology that increase our ability to gather and analyze data. The miniaturization of electronics made motion sensing on mobile phones and wearables possible. Improvements in battery life and low-power chipsets made sensing devices last longer than a day. The introduction of Bluetooth Low Energy Radio made it possible for devices to efficiently connect, and, of course, cloud computing for storing and processing data made everyday sensing conceivable. Much work has been done simply to make sure that the electronics don't melt, which alone is a tremendous task. Some things are technologically easier to sense, steps versus stress or hormones, for instance, and that influences what people choose to keep track of as much as a cultural preoccupation with "healthism" or the "wellness syndrome."[20]

Engineers must contend with the brute facts of circuitry, but they also have their own social imaginations. There are many "visions" circulating within the technology-building community, and these visions inform what eventually makes it to the marketplace. *Ubiquitous computing*, the idea that computers would one day be a part of bodies and environments, not just offices, arose in the 1980s and has been an important idea within technology communities ever since. This idea effectively made "wearability" thinkable. *Persuasive computing* is the idea that computers can "nudge" people to act in particular ways, and this idea, too, helped create common design strategies in wearables. This subfield of computer science also championed *gamification*, or using game techniques to encourage users to perform a certain action. Gamification turns activities into games, such as awarding points or stars for flossing or running, or using more elaborate and sophisticated strategies to reward certain behaviors or actions. Another idea driving the technology industry is social network analysis. New forms of media have been built upon the "six degrees of separation" experiments of the sociologist Stanley Milgram in the 1960s. Facebook, Twitter, and professional networking events alike owe their popularity to the rediscovery of the idea of social networks. Now most activity-tracking apps or devices have social features, for example, to invite friends and family to either compete or support. Networks are not the only way to be social, but they are built into most technical systems because they provide a structured way of representing social relationships that computers can handle.

The Communities

In both sociology and anthropology, the term "community" can sometimes refer to strong reciprocal social or familial relationships and other times evoke a particular geographic place. A "community of practice" refers to a group of people who convene around a common interest.[21] Online forums are called "communities," whether they feature genuine social support or merely appeal to nostalgic notions of community in the service of technology firms' self-interests. Regardless, there are many groups and places where people talk about self-tracking data. We will use "community" in this book to refer to the sets of relationships in which people discuss data, whether loose or tight-knit, and whether located in the same place or not. Sometimes these discussions about data happen with family members. Sometimes they happen with doctors. Sometimes people compare data with their friends or others online. Professional communities of practice, too, have their own ways of shaping how self-tracking data is discussed. Our use of *community* for all these different kinds of relationships builds on Charles Kadushin's definition of a social circle, where people recognize others as a part of the circle even if they do not personally know one another.[22] In social circles, people have a sense of who is and who isn't a part and the unwritten rules of membership.

There are several different communities where self-tracking practices unfold. A significant one is Quantified Self, mentioned earlier. After noticing people around the San Francisco Bay Area taking advantage of the enhanced availability of technology for self-tracking, Gary Wolf and

Kevin Kelly, both *Wired* magazine editors, hosted an initial gathering in Kelly's Pacifica, California, home in 2008. Soon after, Wolf started the website quantifiedself.com. There are now QS "meetups" in 119 cities in 38 countries, and regular international conferences and symposia.[23] The QS community emphasizes self-experimentation, which they sometimes refer to as "n-of-1" studies, where the n, or number of cases in the study, is oneself. At most QS meetings people present their own self-tracking experiences through a "show-and-tell talk," and all speakers are asked to plainly answer three questions: What did you do? How did you do it? What did you learn? Many of these talks are video-recorded and posted on the website for others to see.

One key norm within QS is that people focus their comments on what they know is true for themselves, with the implication that it may not be true for everyone. This grounded conversational style makes room for diversity of beliefs, opinions, positions, and values to flourish, while facilitating mutual learning.[24] Quantified Self is also more than a lead user group. It is evolving as a social arena where people discuss many of the social controversies discussed in this book. Quantified Self uses the conversational style that it encourages among lead users to also facilitate conversations about technology and public health that are difficult to have in communities solely devoted to one professional community or another. Some very real progress in the state of the debates is made there, though not exclusively.

Whitney Boesel, a sociologist and a QS member, designed an excellent diagram that differentiates the larger practices of self-tracking from the QS meetups around the world that have grown out of Wolf and Kelly's first meeting (see figure 1.2). Because people often call self-tracking "quantified self," she calls the larger practices "lowercase quantified self" and the named group "uppercase Quantified Self." Her figure uses a circle to show QS, "the group" as she terms it, within a larger set of social practices and phenomena.

The lower-case term "quantified self" is catchy and has been widely used by journalists, industry pundits, and academics alike to refer to anything and everything that might have to do with self-tracking. Journalists now speak of "quantified self technologies"—the pedometers, sleep trackers and so forth—and the "quantified self movement," by which they often mean the many people who use these products and not the smaller number of participants in QS events. Many claims get made in the name of "the quantified self" about the cultural premium placed on self-optimization.

The problem is that in many instances, the term "quantified self" is used to refer to the exact opposite of what people in the QS community are in fact trying to achieve under that name. These usages are often (but not always) indifferent to Quantified Self community members' concerns, and ignore what they have to say and how they

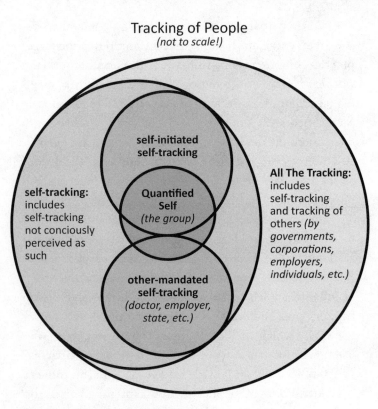

Figure 1.2 Taxonomy of types of tracking.
Source: Whitney Boesel, *The Society Pages.*

define what they are doing. At a QS meeting you won't find people who just swallow the idea that we are all now supposed to optimize ourselves. Instead, you will find people questioning doctors' orders and satisfying their curiosity.

Wolf's own description of the quantified self focuses on discovery, not compliance with a prescribed way of doing things:

> Trackers focused on their health want to ensure that their medical practitioners don't miss the particulars of their condition; trackers who record their mental states are often trying to find their own way to personal fulfillment amid the seductions of marketing and the errors of common opinion; fitness trackers are trying to tune their training regimes to their own body types and competitive goals, but they are also looking to understand their strengths and weaknesses, to uncover potential they didn't know they had. Self-tracking, in this way, is not really a tool of optimization but of discovery.[25]

QS community members all have their own opinion on what "quantified self" really means, and while they do not all match Wolf's, there is something important happening under that name that should not be conflated with these other imaginings about self-tracking. To keep things clear in this book, we will use "self-tracking" when we are talking about the practices and the social phenomenon of people keeping track of themselves. We will say "Quantified Self" to refer to this specific community founded by Wolf and Kelly.

Quantified Self is a significant community, and we will hear more about this group in the pages to come, but it is not the only one in which people wrestle with what data means. Online patient communities have long been a vibrant aspect of the Internet, and now many also incorporate sharing data and include discussion forums where people interpret data together. Some online communities, such as Patients Like Me and Cure Together, ask their members to pool data in order to contribute to greater collective knowledge about conditions and diseases. Other communities have a more social media-style network structure such as we find in hashtag "Twitter chats" like #bcsm (breast cancer social media), #hcsm (healthcare social media), and #hpm (hospice and palliative medicine); in Facebook groups; and on websites organized around particular diseases and conditions. Individual apps and services often provide "social" features, which are designed around social networks or peer-to-peer connections. For example, Coached.me connects potential data-driven life coaches with people who have data and seek advice. These kinds of apps and services typically enable people to share data with a small group or find encouragement or a sense of accountability from others.

There are also communities that form around a specific professional interest in seeing particular visions of self-tracking come into being. These are most visible around health innovation and technology conferences, such as TEDMed, Stanford's Medicine X, O'Reilly Health Foo, HIMSS (Healthcare Information and Management Systems Society), and Health 2.0. They are populated by a mix of entrepreneurs, academics, engineers, venture capitalists, and medical professionals, some with patient advocacy involvement. On the academic side, computer science conferences like Ubicomp, Persuasive Computing, and CHI (Computer-Human Interaction) have studied and developed many of the technology designs now on the market.

Finally, the most important communities are the ones people turn to for help in making sense of their data. People come to understand their data from conversations with others—those understandings do not just come from a vacuum, and they do not just come from online or in-person communities set up for the purpose. Very different conversations about self-tracking data might happen with families, doctors, friends, and other users of self-tracking tools.

Where communities, tools, and practices intersect, we find a set of controversies and social problems that may decide who will ultimately benefit from this phenomenon. In chapter 2, we go deeper into some of the issues at stake. In the subsequent chapters, we delve into how key communities wrestle with these issues through developing new practices and tools.

WHAT IS AT STAKE?
THE PERSONAL GETS POLITICAL

Whether we intentionally self-track, or *are* tracked with or without our consent, our personal data—often of the most intimate and private nature—connects us to wider social systems. Our data contains a virtual, if partial, version of the self—a "data double" living on servers around the world.[1] When it travels, a part of us does, too. In this way, our data has a social life. It is both personal and political at the same time.

Who wants your data, and what do they want to do with it? This chapter outlines the main social dynamics that shape the answer to this question. When self-tracking technologies are discussed in the press, privacy is most often the first concern raised. This makes sense: our privacy is more easily violated when there is more data about us swirling around. But there are many other possible repercussions of self-tracking data, both positive and negative and at individual and societal levels. On the one hand, data from sensing technologies may lead to new forms of discrimination or legitimize negative concepts of the body. On the other hand, individual data, especially when pooled with that of others, could yield discoveries that benefit individuals and communities. We will address privacy last, because understanding these other implications of the technologies helps us understand why privacy is so vital, yet perennially difficult to protect.

Am I Normal?

When people try out an activity tracker for the first time, the first question they often ask is whether their readings are normal. Sometimes "normal" means "what most people do," and at other times, it is used as a synonym for ideal. Many self-tracking tools fail to distinguish between the two. A biomedicalized culture teaches us to measure ourselves in the context of others. This is what science largely does. It measures some phenomenon across a population and creates distributions of people. A "normal" curve, in the mathematical sense, is bell-shaped, with most people being in the middle. Not all medical phenomena have bell-shaped distributions, but nevertheless being outside an imagined "center" is culturally associated with something problematic, perhaps needing medical intervention or requiring self-discipline. However, there might not be an actual problem for any particular individual and the difference between high or low and the center may be simple variation.

This conflation of mathematically normal distribution with "normal" as a kind of ideal gives tremendous power to those who decide what to measure. Many of us live in the sort of society that valorizes "self-improvement" and "taking action." Choosing *not* to do something about a potential problem makes one a double outlier, most definitely "not normal" in the sense of falling short of the cultural ideal of the striving self-improver. Data can burden people with the work of determining whether their data represents ordinary human variation, a physical problem, or a social belief about health and wellness. It is not always possible to distinguish between problems that are pure matters of human biology and problems that become problems because society defines them as "not normal."

Consider the example of activity trackers. Out of the box, most recommend 10,000 steps per day. This is more than double the US average, and, for most people, more than the official recommendation of 150 minutes of activity per week. When someone takes 7,000 steps in a day and sees the app telling her she should really be taking 10,000 steps a day, the question "Am I normal?" is bound to come up. She could decide to accept that "normal" is, in fact, 10,000 steps and accept that she is lacking them.

She might even take more steps, though in reality people only tend to do this while the device is new and interesting. Activity monitors generally do not mention what a "normal" (in the sense of average) step count is for various *types* of people and how this relates to medical conditions or an ideal. What is average for one's age? Fitness level? Medical condition? Should we expect the same number of steps for a seventeen-year-old and a seventy-year-old? The US average is less than in countries where cars are less common, and agricultural peoples around the world take many, many more steps per day than would be considered "normal" or even "ideal" in a Western context. Whether their "normal" is also considered "ideal" is a value-laden judgment as much as a medical assessment of the physical consequences of overwork.

"Am I normal?" then becomes a question about how societies create categories for people—old or young, laborer or desk jockey—and how people then use those categories. One study of workplace-based step counting shows how these categories could evolve as quantification becomes more extensive.[2] A workplace program instituted a team competition for the most steps walked. The competition did not have any long-term effect on activity levels, but it produced a discussion about legitimate reasons to be able or unable to take 10,000 steps a day. Mothers with sick children were excused, while others felt pressure to not let down the group. This was the first time that category—mothers with sick children—was thought about in that light, as the type of situation that would be a "normal" aberration from the social obligation to exercise.

Individual decisions do matter to some extent. A person using an activity tracker could decide that the app designer placed her in the wrong category, perhaps for individuals younger than she was. In fact, when Dawn was recovering from her knee injury, she decided that 3,000 steps was an appropriate level of activity for someone with her type of disability, despite the fact that the manufacturer of her activity tracker kept admonishing her for a "lack" of exercise. However, designs limit the choices we have. While Dawn chose not to take such "encouragement" to get more exercise seriously, she still was subjected to it, forcing her to actively work against the manufacturer's assumption that disability—temporary in her case—is somehow outside the normal range of abilities. In fact, her research suggests the manufacturer was flat-out wrong on this count. In one study, Dawn recruited twenty-nine physically active activity-monitor users, and only two had *not* experienced some type of major injury in recent years.

This leads us to a third possibility. Geography, social commitments, and medical challenges may make 10,000 steps difficult for many people without great sacrifice, but someone might nevertheless *believe* that 10,000 steps *should* be taken every day. A device user may come to see himself instead, through the data and the systems designed to encourage behavior change, as a person who failed. In this situation, the technology acts as a kind of surveillance substitute. It is not the direct gaze of a doctor or other medical person constantly watching, but the recommendations that come with self-tracking tools *sound* authoritative, couched in quasi-medical terms intended for users to internalize as problems that they must solve on their own. Accepting this view of a "failed step-taker" leaves no room for questions about the social situations that create the near impossibility of "active lifestyles" for many people. In most apps, only individual solutions are allowed. "Social" features are not about having a dialogue about public infrastructures and civic conditions that support individual health. They are instead about individuals competing against one another to take more steps. This inward focus, which the philosopher Michel Foucault warned was becoming a central part of contemporary cultures, feeds a sense of inadequacy that creates demand for the next purchase. Believing or rejecting the failed step-taker model is a choice that people can make as technology users, but as long as the technologies are designed in this way, it is not a model that users can simply escape.

The connection between social forces and individual data is complex. The cultural meaning of these categories (failed step-taker, person who can't control her blood glucose levels, the "not-so-biggest" loser of weight), change as there are more kinds of data. Historically, risk categories have been based in demographics, as in the formulation "white women in their mid-40s are at greater risk for X." Risk categories have both social and biological components. For example, it is stressful to be discriminated against within society, and stress increases the chances of some conditions like heart disease. Beliefs about which foods to eat are social and cultural, but they result in people with similar microbiomes, increasingly seen as one key to understanding health. With richer data, the categories that define "people like me" get more complex. Indeed, within Quantified Self there is lively discussion about how, exactly, to move away from asking what is normal toward "what is normal for me?" Anne Wright has argued at QS conferences that using data as a way to compare yourself now to yourself then is a good way to get out of the "am I normal?" trap. Similarly, asking "what has happened to others in my situation?" could be a way of learning from others' experiences in subtler ways. Here, "others in my situation" could be considered across many different parameters.

This is a shift in the style of statistical thinking, the kinds of questions that are legitimate to ask, and the computational ability to answer them. What this shift means for social equity and privacy is an ongoing theme in the pages to come. On one hand, this shift could help the medical "outliers" who have difficult-to-diagnose conditions to work out for themselves what is going on. New advances in *precision medicine* promise a wider scope for tailoring medical decisions based on individuals' data and going beyond traditional diagnostic categories through customized treatment for individual cases. However, as critic Evgeny Morozov points out, if data about our bodies accumulates to levels where "normal for my situation" can be refined with great precision, opting out of data collection might no longer be a viable choice. Opting out will effectively signal having something to hide, with attendant repercussions.[3] While most industrialized countries have clear laws concerning discrimination based on data about gender or race, inferences can be made from nontraditional, unprotected data like social media behavior that can effectively result in discrimination in all but name.

Who Asks the Questions?

It used to be that data was scarce and expensive to collect. Only expert researchers collected data, and only when they had a compelling enough question to answer. Sensors on every phone open up the possibility for people who are not professional researchers to collect data and ask questions about it. For example, Jacqueline Wheelwright, a health coach and an autoimmune disease sufferer, describes how she uses an activity tracker to make sense of what triggers her own disease.[4] By reviewing a year's worth of her

Sensors on every phone open up the possibility for people who are not professional researchers to collect data and ask questions about it.

activity data, she discovered that when she took *too many* steps, her symptoms flared up. Professional medicine had not yet provided evidence about thresholds of activity that could trigger autoimmune symptoms, but she was able to ask whether her flare-ups had to do with activity because she had the data to make that question both conceivable and answerable.

Similarly, Seth Roberts, a self-tracker and psychology professor, ran a series of experiments on his cognitive functioning using a test of reaction times. His data showed him that "there's a lot I didn't/don't know about how my food affects me. Maybe everyone can say that. Unlike almost anyone else, however, I can reduce my ignorance myself. I don't need to rely on experts."[5] Roberts argued that he did not have to mobilize all of his expertise to reduce his ignorance. "Non-experts can discover important things about health. . . . By non-experts I mean people who are not health professionals. People who do not make a living from health research. By discover I mean learn from data for the first time, actually discover—in contrast to learn from an expert. By important I mean stuff that matters to many people." According to Roberts, scientific studies might be valid in a general way, but not always relevant to a particular situation: "Is what those studies found—studying animals, or at best, other humans—true for *you*?[6]

In a data-rich society, the question asker might become you, the person measured in the data, or it might become you in collaboration with a clinical expert or other kind of expert. Here we find an important crossroads. Data could maintain the cultural script that already happens in doctors' offices (i.e., "Have you been measuring your glucose like I asked?") or it could change them, by making different "givens." The word "data," Daniel Rosenberg wrote, is etymologically tied to a notion of "that which is given prior to an argument."[7] Change the givens, and you change the conversation. For example, Katie McCurdy is a graphic designer and self-tracker who drew a graph of symptom severity entirely without numbers.[8] The point of her graph (figure 2.1) was not to render her symptom record "more accurate," but to produce a "given" that could support a conversation with her healthcare providers about her history without having to start at the beginning each time. By asserting these givens, McCurdy opens up the conversation within a frame that bounds the relevant questions. We further explore how these conversations might go, in practice, in chapter 5 on self-tracking and medicine.

Data also has the potential to change who gets a seat at the table when it comes to posing research questions of large populations. In chapter 5 we examine some of the efforts in this area, such as the work of the Cincinnati Children's Chronic Care Network, which pools self-tracking data for use by both clinical researchers and patients' families. Projects in this field each reflect different balances of power between people measured by data and medical

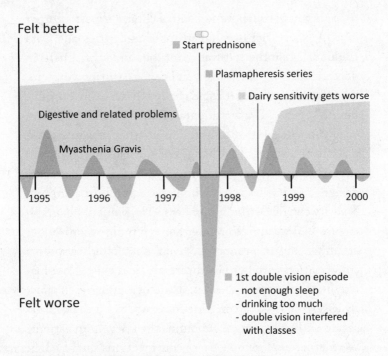

Figure 2.1 Katie McCurdy's health visualization timeline.
Source: Katie McCurdy as adapted by Chris Monson.

professionals. At a gathering of public health researchers and consumer device makers convened by QS, public
health researcher Eric Heckler has argued that science researchers cannot simply hoover up citizen data while ex-
pecting to be able to conduct business as usual.[9] Data for
everyday use is a fundamentally different type of data than
traditional medical data. Such data, from web searches to

mobile devices, can reveal much more than its original purpose for collection. For example, accelerometer data commonly is used to infer steps, but with a different algorithm it can reveal the possible presence of Parkinson's disease. That use of activity trackers is not (yet) validated by clinical studies, but the data is not necessarily clinically irrelevant, either. Yet because it is collected in ongoing ways, it could say something about an individual's personal habits and more day-to-day concerns. Because data has these multiple purposes, and an important connection to personal biography, it does have a potential role in public health research, but people may come to want more of a say in what is done with it.

Two examples illustrate the range of approaches to widening public participation in research. First is Apple's ResearchKit, a technology that enables medical researchers to collect cell phone data from people who opt in to participate in medical research. While ResearchKit facilitates public participation in medical research, at the Quantified Self Public Health Forum some participants complained that this design choice puts the public squarely in the role of data donor by preventing people who do not have institutional review board (IRB) ethics clearance from conducting research. While this rule is likely to protect iPhone users from unethical research, advocates of patient-driven research are concerned that this could also exclude citizen scientists, people outside of established research institutions and centers, from asking questions. Citizen scientists have played a vital role in learning about diseases neglected by institution-based medical research, as in the early days of HIV/AIDS and chronic fatigue syndrome. Their exclusion comes with the social and scientific cost of rocks left unturned. Second, at the opposite end of the spectrum, is PublicLab.org, a group that supports grassroots research agendas for environmental health, and the grassroots development of data-gathering tools necessary to answer environmental health-related questions. Grassroots science experiences challenges in terms of establishing scientific validity and social legitimacy. There remains controversy over whether individual self-tracking projects can in and of themselves be scientifically valid, and thus contribute to our collective scientific knowledge on their own terms, as opposed to just being part of larger data collection efforts. Historians Lorraine J. Daston and Peter Galison show that the idea that scientific practice must be separate from the individual observer to be unbiased was first seen in the nineteenth century when the need arose for "collective empiricism" across many different researchers.[10] Today, Ian Eslick, a QS participant with a doctorate from MIT, builds tools to conduct scientific research on the self. He wouldn't say "let's drop objectivity" because people collect and analyze their own data. Instead, he advocates for a return to this pre-nineteenth-century idea that the scientist can be a disciplined observer of her own experience: "Science is really about repeatability, about process, about discipline, about characterization, about controlling noise, and there are lots of different mechanisms that we can pull together to tell a story or inform a decision."[11] In other words, scientific proof need not be the only reason to seek answers to our questions.

If there is broader participation in asking questions, will this change the kinds of questions asked? It has historically been the case that people with more diverse backgrounds and different perspectives think of questions that established researchers do not. Diversity can be particularly important when established research is in a state of "problem closure," a situation where the participants believe they already know what the loop of facts and action are, and any new facts that do not fit within that loop are ignored. Indeed, we can see evidence of problem closure when "behavior change" does not happen through activity trackers, and yet new versions of those technologies do not change the fundamental approach to the problem. When established ways of thinking become pervasive throughout a society, simply changing the actors doesn't necessarily bring new perspectives. Our sense is that there still is diversity of ideas about health and the body despite pervasive biomedicalization, and in chapter 3 we discuss what some of those ideas look like. Whether this diversity can be mobilized to organize a broader social movement, or whether self-tracking practices prove too individualistic to lead to collective action, is an open question.

Public Health Outcomes

Larry Smarr, labeled by *The Atlantic* as "the measured man," is the director of a computer science research institute who conducted a series of elaborate tests on his intestinal microbiome. Even though he felt fine and could not report any symptoms to his doctor, his data told him that he was decidedly *not* fine. At the 2012 QS Conference he argued, "This idea that you can just feel what is going on inside of you, that is just so epistemologically false. You just can't do it."[12]

In Smarr's view, data is about seeing what we cannot see or feel otherwise. Seeing more phenomena, across more people, holds the potential for better public health outcomes if used in the right way. Medical practitioners and health technology developers also think about the promise of better health outcomes, but with an eye to medical compliance, rather than new discoveries. Unlike the critical theorists inspired by Foucault and concerned about the power held by medicalized normativity, these actors unabashedly look to self-tracking tools and practices as a way to encourage patients to comply with treatments and regimens, follow recommended guidelines for healthy eating and exercise, and manage chronic conditions more effectively. While we take the critical scholarship seriously, the clinical view is not an unreasonable one. It argues better decisions are made, physiologically speaking, when standard medical knowledge—the outcome of collective empiricism—is disseminated through the use of self-tracking devices. Technologies have the capacity, in effect, to deliver medical advice at scale in more areas of daily life, and with more precise control over the context in which they are delivered.

Does this actually work? Are people actually physically healthier through more extensive use of self-tracking technology? We wrestle with this question in chapter 5, but the short answer is that it the jury is out, and it depends on whom you ask. An exchange at a session on self-tracking data at the Medicine X conference at Stanford University summarizes the complexity of the issue. One panelist claimed, "Data leads to knowledge and knowledge leads to change." A woman in the audience stood up and said, "As a career-long psychologist, I can tell you that if that were true there would be no need for psychologists."

Many established programs for self-improvement, whether a diet, a financial plan, or a productivity program, do start with data that brings to light patterns of behavior through some form of tracking. But, simply knowing (and agreeing) that a behavior is healthy or unhealthy may not be enough to change it. In fact, one of our own interviewees, a public health researcher, laughed at the short-term feed-back loops assumed to be effective in self-tracking devices: "If that behavior is part of your core identity, it will take at least four years to shift it." However, the claim that "data leads to knowledge leads to change" is a seductive one for companies that are in the business of finding "moments of opportunity," as Elizabeth Bierbower, an executive at the healthcare group Humana, puts it. People like Bierbower see opportunities to "deliver the right information at the right time, through the right intervention"[13] through real-time knowledge of one's activities. It seems like it should work, and it certainly appeals to insurers in terms of costs. "Real time knowledge," however, might be more difficult to make meaningful in practice. Simplistic, short-term mod-els of health behavior change also might not withstand the weight of social complexity.

Why turn to technology and data, as opposed to other forms of communication, to deliver medical advice at all? Annemarie Mol's research suggests that the inclination to deliver medical advice through technology has to do with how healthcare as an institutional practice has evolved.[14] She argues that Western healthcare systems have tried to facilitate patient choice, but "choice" went hand in hand with the bureaucratization of healthcare, turning medical decision making into a kind of algorithm or recipe. Blood glucose too high? The protocol says do X, but not Y. With greater patient choice, and standardization across medical systems, now any doctor the patient chooses will also say do X (but not Y), because that is what the clinical evidence shows. The problem, Mol points out, is that the work of caring means going off script and giving nonstandard advice that takes into account the patient's personal situation and priorities. She calls this the difference between the logic of care and the logic of choice. In the logic of care, keeping someone's glucose stable means having a clinical discussion about, say, whether it is worthwhile to let the blood glucose occasionally go low in order to do things that make life worth living, like hiking. In the logic of choice, technologies or clinicians offer a simple cutoff point, and alarms go off when the threshold has been reached. While not having to go into the clinic can be freeing, if the freedom to choose is only about choosing forms of protocol delivery, she argues it ultimately is not a meaningful choice.

The bureaucratization of healthcare delivery makes it easier for technologies to substitute for types of interventions and emphasizes certain market logics. Long-standing bureaucracies in the private sector are particularly vulnerable to "disruption," or competing with smaller upstarts that deliver a different kind of product.[15] Chapter 5 describes some of the key players in the health and wellness technologies markets who have set themselves the agenda of "disrupting medicine." Whether positive public health outcomes come to pass through technology adoption depends on the practices that technologies are actually displacing, and whether technologies are being used as a substitute, or supplement, for care.

Increasing reliance on self-serve technologies effectively shifts labor costs to patients. There is an important distinction to make between expanding individual control, such as enabling more people to interpret their own data, and austerity-driven *individuation*, where matters that were once taken care of by social institutions through paid labor are foisted onto people and their families, who now must do it as unpaid labor, with only some help from technology, regardless of whether they wanted to take it on themselves. The promise of individuals "taking control," particularly valorized in the United States, and touted by the healthcare devices industry, may very well be a burden disguised as empowerment.

Throughout this book, we encourage readers to ask questions about the healthcare institutions in which they find themselves. Is the technology you are being asked to use really going to improve your health, or is it shifting the administrative or healthcare labor onto you? If you are using it voluntarily, does it help you make *sense* of the situation, or does the rich data just go off to someone else while you get an unhelpful number? Is it a protocol delivery device, or are there places where actual care, in Annemarie Mol's sense, can be found?

The promise of individuals "taking control" may very well be a burden disguised as empowerment.

Who Has Access to Data?

Access to self-tracking data ultimately is about who has the right to analyze data and benefit from the answers. It would be easy to see data access as a problem only geeks or hypochondriacs have. But consider the case of Dana Lewis and Scott Leibrand, who are provoking an important public discussion about what level of access people should be able to get to their own data. Lewis and Leibrand used their admittedly geeky skills to connect Dana's continuous glucose monitor with her implanted insulin pump.[16] As someone with Type 1 diabetes, Dana was particularly concerned about nighttime hypoglycemia. Low blood-sugar levels do not wake up people with diabetes, but they can kill them in their sleep. Like many people managing Type 1, Dana was well aware of the patterns between her eating and exercise and her blood glucose readings, and she adjusted her insulin dosage accordingly. These patterns, she and Scott found, were regular enough that they could be built into an algorithm, adjusted over time by Dana, based on what she would normally do while awake. The algorithm they developed "closes the loop" by using data from the continuous glucose monitor to trigger a dose of insulin. This approximated what Dana would have done while she was awake, reducing her risk of nighttime hypoglycemia. Access to data at a level deeper than just being able to see it on a screen mattered greatly to Dana. To write this algorithm,

Dana had to switch to an older model of continuous glucose monitor, because the newer models prohibit access to the data outside the company's proprietary readout.

While Dana and Scott's work is not without controversy, it points to the importance of people having access to their own data. Even if this is not a task that most people would care to take on, user-driven innovation in medical technologies is something many people stand to benefit from, and it relies on data access. In response to numerous inquiries about the method, the duo launched the Open Artificial Pancreas System to share their techniques with others. Some would like to see their algorithm validated through clinical trials and approved by regulators, while others wish these two could distribute their work through other means. While there are reasonable debates about the best means of dissemination, it is clear that more people could benefit from user-driven innovation like this and that data access matters.

Many, but not all, companies recognize that there will always be uses for the data they produce beyond what they support. There are two ways companies can accommodate these extra uses. One is by providing a data download button for direct use by end users. The other is by building an application programming interface, or API, so that other software providers can retrieve data on users' behalf.

While seemingly technical, this is another important area where the personal becomes political. "APIs are an opinion about the data worth having," Aaron Coleman, founder of Fitabase, noted at the 2015 Quantified Self Public Health Symposium. Coleman knows this problem more than most. His company facilitates permissions and handoffs between Fitbit users and medical researchers, and he has worked with Fitbit to adapt their API so that the data offered is useful for research. Companies only pay the extra cost of supplying and maintaining APIs if they have a sense for what individuals, public health researchers, or other companies want to do with the data. Building a data download button is much cheaper than building an API, but decisions about what to offer still have to be made. Asking for "all the raw data" does not help companies offer it—there are too many decisions to be made about what "raw" means in practice. Dawn attempted to clean heart rate data from her activity tracker data to understand when her elevated heart rate could not be attributed to exercise. She was able to do it using data already "cooked" into steps, but had no hope of doing it using "raw" accelerometer data, not being the type of person who has a steps-conversion algorithm on hand. When individual end users have a concrete sense of the kind of data most useful to them, they stand a better chance of influencing companies to provide it. Of course, companies that believe they exclusively own people's data or see competitive advantage in hiding the method they used to process it will be less persuaded by such arguments.

Who Profits?

We have discussed only briefly how data access matters, and through the rest of the book we will show in more detail what access means to people pushing the boundaries of self-tracking, the industry, and medical practice. There is one final point to be made about why data access matters, and that has to do with market structures. Companies go out of business, and change their products, regularly. Without data download or APIs, users could be locked into a newly defunct service, and not ever get their data back. Some self-trackers call these companies "data roach motels," in the sense that the data can enter, but it can never leave. Whether a market with high switching costs for consumers can still be described as a competitive market is a question that regulatory bodies will have to face if the industry does not demonstrate that it can support data portability.

That there are potential concerns about fair market behavior reminds us that there are sizeable sums of money at stake in self-tracking data. The notion that data is "monetizable," or the new oil, is a fundamental belief motivating many companies and funders behind self-tracking technologies. The economic value of data puts limits on what companies are willing to share with other companies, end users, or researchers. It also stokes fantasies about the money that can be made with ever-greater data stockpiles—fantasies that may or may not be realistic. We talk more about this idea in chapter 4, "Self-Tracking and the Technology Industry."

Data as an economic asset is an important factor in public deliberation about how much of life should be open to commodification. When you are not paying the full cost of a service, and that service is run by a for-profit company, chances are fairly good that your data, or your attention, is what is being sold. Surveillance studies scholar David Phillips and his coauthors called this phenomenon the "self as commodity." Similarly, Brad Millington, a sports and health sociologist, has commented that "interactive, customizable technologies provide new means for monitoring, discussing, and indeed commodifying health and fitness."[17] The virtual self represented in data is being sliced and diced into decontextualized parts, and bought and sold. Many other aspects of life have similarly become commodities when once they were not (land, water, and labor are three examples), but usually societies place limits on what is and is not subject to commodity logic. What kind of limits should be placed on how data is used and circulated is a matter of controversy. For many people, it is one thing for companies to have access to personal information in order to be able to deliver a useful product, but it is quite another for that company to then also sell that data. Even with identifying information stripped out, that data is still a part of ourselves. At some point, we all draw a line at which we say that data about ourselves, which is really a representation of each of us as an individual, is incompatible with that sort of activity. When that line is crossed, we might start to suspect that privacy violations are occurring. In the next and final section, we will show how privacy objections have everything to do with how representations of the self intersect with a commodified world.

Privacy Is a Moving Target

So far, we have seen how some companies buy and sell data generated from your body because legally it is theirs to sell, even though it pertains to you. Meanwhile, participate in any QS meeting and you might find people complaining about companies that refuse to help customers understand what went into calculating "sleep quality score" or other measures, because they do not want to reveal a proprietary algorithm. To this list we could add the discussions of making it a crime to reidentify anonymous data that have emerged in the United Kingdom in response to the National Health Service's plans to centralize and share patients' records there.

These situations all have two key elements in common. First, privacy is not protected simply because names and addresses have been stripped away from the data. Not only can these be reinserted, but also there are clear cases where a sense of invasion or violation is present without individuals being named or targeted directly. We can feel violated without direct reidentification because our expectations of privacy have to do with what philosopher Helen Nissenbaum calls "contextual integrity." When information is collected about us, we have a reasonable set of assumptions and understandings of what that data is for, and who is involved in that particular context.[18] Unexpected changes break the assumptions we made about that context, yielding a sense of violation. Because privacy is so dependent on the specific context, we cannot say that this or that data is especially "private." What makes data "private" is the lineup of people or institutions "in context" for issues related to the data and the body to which the data refers. You might not share with your doctor the fight you had with your husband because it is too personal and out of context, but you might not share with your husband what you share with your doctor and, de facto, your insurance company, for exactly the same reason.

This does not mean that institutions are off the hook for privacy because it is "all relative." Quite the opposite. To take privacy seriously requires an even higher bar for being sensitive to the social contexts in which institutions work, and a willingness to trace out the likely data flows. Illegible, changeable terms-of-service documents are spectacularly context-insensitive, designed to absolve organizations of responsibility. Such documents do not meet that higher bar for contextual integrity, even if they might abide by the letter of the law. Throughout the rest of the book, you will encounter examples of ways that companies do (or do not) maintain contextual integrity.

These examples involve differing beliefs about ownership, and how those differences break contextual integrity. In popular understanding, ownership is usually thought of as binary—you either own something, or somebody else does. Data, however, is never created by just one party. Steps data comes into existence because there is a person who takes the steps, and because there is a person or company that has designed technology to represent those steps as data. So whose data is it? Anthropologist Bill Maurer has suggested that when it comes to sorting out ownership claims, data is better thought about using principles that we apply to kinship (i.e., how people are related to one another) rather than the principles we use for commodities exchange.[19] In our steps example, we could think of the steps data as effectively the "child" of the interaction between you and the activity-tracker company. You could not have made that data alone, but neither could the company.

With children come a bundle of rights and responsibilities that are shared between the parents and among the parents and child. These rights and responsibilities are enduring—only in the most extreme circumstances can they be signed away. Could we reimagine the rights and responsibilities for data in a similar way, when self-tracking data is born of a user and the company who makes the technology? Given that self-tracking data is part of the intimate representation of a person's life story, the comparison to kinship is a reasonable one. A "virtual self" has been born.

Thinking about market relationships like buyer and seller for data is quite different than the rights and responsibilities of kinship. If data is only ever a commodity, then those responsibilities among parties are over once it is bought, sold, or exchanged for a service. This sense of equitable commodity transaction, where both parties got what they want, is what companies rely on when they subsequently monetize personal data. Such transactions are essentially saying, "Nothing we do with the data pertains to you after the exchange." Many conflicts over the proper use of data stem from the way that data as a commodity cuts off the enduring stakes that people have in the data about themselves. This commodity logic applied to data has little room for the idea that representations of you remain a part of you and have continuing consequences for you. There is only so much of oneself that a person can alienate away. Recognizing people's rights as the "parents" of their own data is not incompatible with market exchange of data, but requires valuing aspects of life outside of markets, too. We could go so far as to say that personal data is *both* a market commodity and a nonmarketable "child" that creates for us responsibilities toward one another.

The commoditization of data should concern every-one worried about the role of commoditization of life more generally and people who want more robust privacy protections. Protecting privacy beyond companies' assurances relies on a notion of more meaningful obligations to the data subjects—the people the data refers to—after an exchange has occurred. This is a more extensive sense of obligation than a strictly market view would allow.

In the next chapter, we take up the specific practices of self-tracking and the different ways that people try to make tracking work for their own goals and contexts.

MAKING SENSE OF DATA

This chapter looks at creative uses of self-tracking. It examines what people go through when they take an off-the-shelf product and make it work for their own situation or purposes. Data is a strange product in the sense that it often reveals more than its designers intended, yet less than is required to be useful. For example, home electricity monitors inadvertently paint a picture of when someone is home or away. Yet how much can a single electricity monitor really say about whether you are an efficient user of energy overall, or what you can do about your usage level if it is high? That might require more data, a different calculation with the data you have, or further research about the problem. To get something out of data, many people find that they have to tinker to make data suit their own contexts and purposes. Often this means combining an off-the-shelf sensor product with some other form of tracking.

Those of us who do not share the patience for extended exploring and tinkering can still learn from practices developed by people who do enjoy that. When Dawn broke her kneecap, she drew on what she had learned from others in order to figure out the best way to keep track of her medicines. That sharing of ideas helped her not have to deal with some apps' inappropriate settings that she found annoying. There is a near infinite diversity in what people do with data, and we cannot show it all here. Our goal is to describe some common practices, highlight the very real skills involved in going "off label" for self-tracking tools, and share some of the potential payoffs of doing so.

People gather at QS meetups to discuss what they could do with their data and the pitfalls that they find. Sometimes people get stuck when trying to make sense of their data, and people in QS often share new things to try out and suggestions for getting unstuck. For that reason, most of the examples here come from the people we encountered by being involved in QS. We recognize, though, that these are practices that many people can do, and many already do them without thinking of themselves as "self-trackers."

While each project is different, here we look more closely at five common styles or purposes for self-tracking: (1) monitoring and evaluating, (2) eliciting sensations, (3) aesthetic curiosity, (4) debugging a problem, and (5) cultivating a habit. We provide examples of what people do in each, along with suggestions about the practical aspects of tracking in that way, for two reasons. The first is to enable you to try these things out for yourself, which involves considerations and pitfalls that others have found that you won't find in the device manuals. We do this in a spirit similar to the QS show-and-tell talks, in that these are ideas we have seen work for other people, or ourselves, but they might not work for you, and they certainly do not aspire to become "best known methods" or a scientific gold standard. Even if you have no interest in trying self-tracking out for yourself, it is still useful to see the dilemmas that people face when they conduct these projects in order to see the creativity that many people bring to them. People who self-track are not, as the critic Evgeny Morozov charges, unthinkingly following whatever computers tell them to do, or allowing technologies to substitute for feelings and emotions.[1]

Tracking to Monitor and Evaluate

Most commercially available self-tracking devices are designed for evaluation and monitoring. Did I take enough steps today? Have I spent my time productively? Such questions imply a target or goal, where both the problem and solution are already known—walk more steps or be more productive. In this form of self-tracking, the data is treated as if its significance is self-evident—more steps are better and improved productivity is good. Once people have settled on what to track, the numbers are collected to make visible a gap between what was actually done and some desired target. Upon further reflection, of course, people might adjust what they track.

Quantified Self participant Amelia Greenhall did several tracking projects in this way. She noticed that her self-tracking experiments made her feel like she was giving herself gold stars for doing the things that made her happy, so she created a paper wall chart to literally give herself gold stars and to track the small actions that she accomplished. "Tracking these things," she said, "make[s] me do more." Her method highlighted *what* she did, not when or how frequently she did it. Seeing a total number—fifteen gold stars, say, for the fifteen times that she went for a short run—gave Greenhall a greater sense of self-accomplishment than focusing on the lack of a run for any particular day. Greenhall also considered the time scales that mattered to her. For someone who has never run before, fifteen runs is a lot, and seeing fifteen shiny gold stars in a row is more encouraging than seeing the same number charted over a number of months.[2]

Like Greenhall, many self-trackers learn how to make judgments about which data is most appropriate for which goal, and whether the gap between reality and goal is one that even needs closing. Many self-trackers think of this process as a kind of feedback loop, a term from computer science for a system that generates information and then adjusts in response to that information. The feedback loop is not on autopilot. Some may consider Greenhall's tracking method imprecise, but both her choice to use stars as opposed to recording the length of the run and her choice not to include a time stamp for her runs were deliberate and communicated something more important for her project than more precise measures could.

Practical Considerations When Tracking to Evaluate

Some activities are inherently more difficult to track than others. For example, food tracking is popular, but it is also one of the most difficult forms of tracking because portion sizes and exact contents of foods are hard to estimate. Some apps solve this problem by preloading their systems with nutritional information about processed foods, but this discourages eating fresh foods. It is worth trying to find the simplest way of collecting data that suits the purpose of the tracking project. This might mean reflecting on the underlying goals more deeply. For food tracking, precise calorie information is harder to collect, but precision only matters if you have a specific calorie goal in mind for a particular reason. Measures that are qualitative (capturing qualities) or subjective (your own opinion) may be just as useful. A common practice is to take a picture of your food just before eating, which can track qualities like color, freshness, and portion size without having to look up a calorie count. This could just as easily record change over time as a calorie count. If your goal is to eat healthier meals, then simply keeping track of your own subjective rating for each meal might be easiest (i.e., *healthful*, *neutral*, *indulgent*).

Similarly, numbers can discourage people when they carry symbolic meaning. Looking at one's weight can be so disheartening that weighing yourself can be counterproductive.[3] One self-tracker in the Portland, Oregon, QS meetup figured out that if she switched the units to something unfamiliar (pounds to kilos, or vice versa) she could track changes without focusing on the numbers that bother her.

Some users become so used to activity monitoring that when they forget their activity trackers they feel like exercise doesn't "count." Many sensor-based devices do not allow users to enter an estimate or correct the sensor when it is clearly wrong. This means that weekly averages and other calculations are affected when users forget to wear the device. When Dawn was helping to prototype Data Sense, a tool for working with data, she heard extensive complaints within QS about this common constraint, and worked to enable users to enter a guesstimate after the fact, which might reflect the situation more accurately than a precisely recorded zero. This problem only occurs when the tracking is automated, as with sensors.

Self-Tracking to Elicit Sensations

When people elicit sensations through tracking, they shuttle between observing physical signals felt in the body and observing the recordings of them. Working between the two, they better define or feel a phenomenon. The data becomes a "prosthetic of feeling," something to help us sense our bodies or the world around us. These senses can become uncannily reliable. Sociologist Whitney Boesel tells the story of a woman who came to develop a stronger sense of when she was ovulating through repeated use of at-home ovulation monitors—strong enough, in fact, that she got better at predicting her ovulation cycle than certain kinds of tests.[4] In another project, a relatively fit and healthy man in his midthirties, living on the US West Coast, monitored his glucose levels in order to understand how his body was responding to sugar. He did not have diabetes, but sugar affects all bodies, each a bit differently. He took a moment after doing the glucose test to mentally make note of how he felt. Energetic? Calm? Full? Shaky? He noted what else was going on, such as, say, a stressful meeting or exercise. He was not trying to maintain an optimal glucose level, but was using the data to develop ideas about how his body responded to sugar.

The data becomes a "prosthetic of feeling," something to help us sense our bodies or the world around us.

Sometimes a sensor need not even be involved. Robin Barooah, an early participant in QS, recorded how much energy he had after each meal using a subjective score. The recording was really a moment of pause, designed to re-sensitize him to the physical signals that used to help him maintain weight, but he had grown desensitized to. He said, "Diets don't work . . . [so] the conclusion I came to was that maybe I could re-learn to regulate my weight. And by 'learn,' I don't mean have a system that I practice, but that I can teach my body to regulate my weight again in a way that it had done [before]."[5] His method was not concerned with what the psychology or physiology about weight loss said, but it served his goal of re-learning how to experience satiety, and he did in fact lose weight. This form of tracking, perhaps more strongly than the others, is often what people have in mind when they say their tracking is connected to mindfulness. Through the numbers they become aware of their bodily states.

These types of projects can generate ideas about causes and effects, which sometimes lead to a hypothesis. The late quantified self pioneer Seth Roberts was fond of saying that you can't falsify a hypothesis you don't have.[6] The project on blood glucose put the man who did it in a position to develop hypotheses about the interaction between stress and sugar, for instance. This bodily awareness he developed could also lead to new ideas about what the body is capable of experiencing. Former *Wired* magazine editor Kevin Kelly has called these technology-mediated sensations "exosenses," to refer to how technology can enhance our ability to sense our bodies and our environments.[7] For example, a German research team created a belt that intermittently vibrates in response to following directions. After a while the wearers learned to intuit where north was without the help of the belt, and, in the words of the project team, to "feel space."[8] Here technology is not replacing awareness, but redirecting it, extending sensations in new ways.

Practices for Tracking to Elicit Sensations

Trial and error is often integral to this style of tracking. For example, we have seen that many people who track their mood find it necessary to rotate through different software, or devise their own system, as their understanding of mood becomes more nuanced. In the beginning of such a project, recording happy or sad using a scale from 1 to 10 might work. As awareness becomes more nuanced, a different recording strategy might be needed. Sadness is qualitatively not the same as anger, and differentiating among different conditions of "not happy" may become important.

As with other forms of tracking, purpose matters for deciding what data to collect. If the goal is to detect a slide into depression, then how many low mood scores have been recorded and for how long might matter more than accurately describing those moods. Conversely, qualitative descriptions (happy, pensive, excited) could paint a better picture of the range of moods experienced.

An important, if tricky, aspect to tracking without the aid of sensors (i.e., manual tracking) is determining whether the data entered refers to right now, the past few hours, or a whole day. Most eliciting-sensations projects track what is being felt "right now," but this need not be the case. Often people say they are having a good or a bad day, so in our mood example, it would make sense to start out by entering "happy" or "7" as an indication of the day as a whole. If that stops feeling like the best way to capture moods, then that itself could be a way of learning about how long moods last.

How data like moods are labeled communicates what is within the sphere of conceivability. Some tracking apps use enum, which are preset labels for a category. They might include as the options for mood "happy," "anxious," or "depressed." Some self-trackers prefer to use instead non-medical language that has meaning for them. A single label may suffice for some people's self-tracking goals. Others, however, might benefit from a second or third descriptor for a point in time (we can be both "happy" and "anxious"). What matters is that you use labels that fit with the kinds of feelings or sensations you are trying to understand or experience.

In practice, tracking to elicit feelings or awareness often means keeping at bay the urge to judge. Eliciting sensations can help in developing hypotheses, but avoiding filtering data to match the emerging explanation can be difficult. Note that eliciting sensations is the opposite of the process of medical diagnosis, which often works through the rapid elimination of possibilities. In this style of tracking, hypotheses and solutions are put on pause in order to develop the fullest possible physically embodied sense of what could be going on.

Aesthetic Curiosity

Just as Man Ray made sculptures, paintings, and photographs out of physical models of mathematical calculations in the 1930s, some artists are now using personal data as material for creating visual forms. One artist, Laurie Frick, converted the GPS data from her phone into collage-like images of abstract patterns (see figure 3.1). Frick uses data as a texture upon which to build art, not as science or evidence. Similarly, sculptor Stephen Cartwright gives shape to material through tracked data. He has recorded his exact latitude, longitude, and elevation every hour of every day since 1999, and combines this data with other variables to make sculptural representations. The resulting art is abstract, largely about the visual form.[9] Cartwright's images weren't meant as aids to help interpret or analyze data, yet his art shows that such visualizations can help a person tell stories, nonetheless.

Satisfying aesthetic curiosity is similar to eliciting sensations in some ways. In Rob Walker's MFA class in design at the School of Visual Arts in New York City, students embark on specific exercises in "practicing paying attention" to strengthen the ability to see what is overlooked.[10]

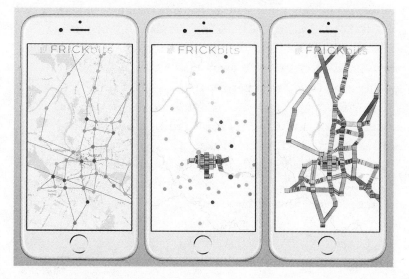

Figure 3.1 Laurie Frick's FrickBits.
Source: Laurie Frick.

Walker considers himself a partisan in what he calls the "war against seeing." He is concerned that companies occupy every corner of people's attention, leading people to interpret the world on terms invented by the companies. To train themselves to see differently Walker's students go on scavenger hunts for the kinds of objects that corporations are less likely to call our attention to. These objects begin to seem much more common after the start of the project. The processes of noticing, counting, and recording into a collage or other visual form make the students more aware of objects' prevalence, changing their perspectives.

Some projects create data to render a specific image. Users of tracking software for running and bicycling have been known to make "drawings" with their data by choosing routes that have particular shapes. Building on that practice, Daniela Rosner and her team at the University of Washington made Trace, an app that generates walking routes based on digital sketches people create and annotate. One person can draw a heart, which the app then maps onto street directions, creating a secret message that the recipient unlocks by walking.[11]

Practical Considerations for Aesthetic Projects

Aesthetic projects are not limited to artists. Experiencing the visual aspects of data can be an important way for people to explore their daily lives beyond data's literal meaning. For example, someone who has been taking pictures of his food every day might have the materials for a collage on his hands. There might be some visually satisfying aspect to these images if assembled in a new way. Even if there is nothing particularly visually compelling, visualizations of data might become interesting as a way of narrating personal biographies. "Charlie," for example, recorded the cardinal direction he was facing every minute, and did not have a particularly strong sense of why he did this other than "for fun." Yet, when people asked him to explain the data, he was able to revisit particular memories, and tell his personal story in a new way.[12]

For those interested in doing a visual project like this but who are not trained in art, it is important to remember that conceptually satisfying work does not require polished graphic design. Conversely, aesthetic sophistication can hide an absence of meaning.[13] What matters is what you see in your personal data, not what others might see. In fact, working with one's own data can also be a good way to start developing data visualization skills, as you are more likely to understand the full context of what it means in relation to some other data set. Rob Walker's list of "20 ways to win in the war against seeing," drawn up as part of his School of Visual Arts course, is an excellent way to get you thinking about the kinds of data that could be interesting to collect.[14]

Debugging a Problem

Debugging is a process in computer programming to figure out why a system is not working as planned. There are many times when a medical diagnosis alone cannot specify triggers for symptoms. Allergies, migraines, asthma, fatigue, and sleep issues are all such situations. Triggers vary from person to person and finding them often can only be done outside a clinical setting. For the unhelpfully diagnosed (as in, "yes you have migraines, but, no, we don't know what triggers yours"), and the entirely undiagnosed, data can be a particularly powerful tool. It can also be used as an effective tool for other sorts of problems, like figuring out why electricity bills are so high, or why financial budgets do not reflect spending patterns in practice. The purpose of debugging is often to figure out how to solve a problem or what brings relief, not necessarily to find the underlying biomedical cause. Debugging is often not a set of "clean" experiments as presented in scientific publications, but then again the purpose is not to publish but to find relief—to debug, not prove.

Anne Wright's story is particularly telling of how useful data can be. She is a former NASA roboticist who used her scientific skills to debug her medical issue. Wright grew too sick to work because of—in her words—"the vague stuff that makes it hard to do what you care about in life [but] that comes up negative on all the tests."[15] The issue was suspected to be gastrointestinal, and she went to multiple specialists without receiving a helpful diagnosis or understanding of the triggers or causes of her problem.

Wright turned to her debugging skills. With the Mars Rovers she worked on, "when something went wrong, there was no flow chart of diagnostics leading to categories of malfunction and repair instructions, such as you would expect with standardized products like cars or refrigerators. Instead, we had to compare expectations against observations."[16] She began to do the same for her body, taking pictures of what she was eating and experimenting with heart-rate sensors. At her doctor's cautious suggestion, she restricted herself to an Ayurveda-prescribed diet. Tracking the consequences of this diet, among many other things, made her realize that the flare-ups happened when one of three ingredients, all in the nightshade family, were used. After reading about other people's experiences and attending lectures in biology, Wright began to understand the biomedical reasoning for why she was having her reaction.

Wright's experience is an important reminder that diagnostic categories and tests are designed for the people who fall in the center of the bell curve, not outliers. Emerging diagnoses, like chronic fatigue syndrome, "you have to fight to get."[17] Medical professionals raise doubts about the veracity of patient stories when they do not fit within current knowledge or protocols that are designed around the center of the bell curve. Through patient advocacy, conditions like chronic fatigue syndrome are now at least partially accepted within medicine. There are some medical problems, like Wright's, that are too rare to gain acknowledgment through advocacy. However, in her case there were enough people who could communicate their own similar problems, which helped her make sense of hers. Not everyone will be lucky enough to find a nonmedical resolution, but Wright thankfully did. She shares her story publicly to show that it is possible to make sense of a medical issue precisely when you might need it most— when others cannot. In fact, data has proved so effective in her being able to get on with her life that, alongside growing active in the QS community, she changed her career. Wright went on to start BodyTrack, a project to help people learn to become peer "data coaches."

Practical Considerations for Debugging

Anne Wright served as Dawn's "peer data coach" for a short time. While there is no single way to debug yourself, our suggestions reflect what Dawn learned from that experience. For debugging, there seem to be three factors worth recording: the symptoms themselves; the things that could be possible culprits, triggers, or causes; and the things that could possibly bring relief. It can be useful to start by creating a data set that records what else is going on at the time the symptoms start, or just before. This uses tracking to narrow the list of possible culprits, such as certain foods, lack of sleep, or stressful days. Similarly, using language to describe as closely as possible the sensations felt, not necessarily jumping to medical language or explanations, could preserve data that might prove important later on.

With a list of possible culprits and ideas about what might bring relief, one can start asking how these are best tracked. Manually? With a sensor or a smartphone? Quantifiedself.com maintains an extensive list of tools and their descriptions. Be sure to look into the specifics of the data a device provides. If you really only care about, say, sleep duration, and the manufacturer only gives you bed times and wake times, that is not the device for you. Also check that there is some way of bringing that data together with any manually tracked data (usually through a data export feature). Manual tracking will also involve deciding for yourself what form the data should take. We provide some considerations for doing this at the end of this chapter.

Some people simply develop a feel for how long it makes sense to track, and when they have learned all they can from one method. Others draw from experiment-driven research to clarify causes and effects. Mark Drangsholt is a University of Washington professor who teaches evidence-based medicine and who suffers from a heart rhythm disorder. He has argued that while many of his colleagues in medicine believe self-tracking to be of a "low level of [scientific] evidence, I don't know if that's really true."[18] Drangsholt advocated for case-crossover design as a way of improving the scientific quality of evidence from a single case. It divides up an individual person's data into "control" data collected during one's normal routine, "exposure" data about potential triggers collected before symptoms, and "hazard" data collected during symptoms. In Drangsholt's case, poor sleep, more than one glass of wine, and public speaking were some of the "exposures" that increased the "hazard" of having a heart incident. This allows for comparison, albeit over time, not across people, and enables formal calculation of the risk of symptoms occurring upon exposure. Through this, Drangsholt found evidence that satisfied him both as a scientist and as the person looking to avoid triggering his heart disorder.

Case-crossover design involves some statistical crunching, and the method can be found online. Another type of testing, *A/B/A/B testing*, alternates treatment and nontreatment periods, so that the difference before and after an intervention becomes clearer. Here the self-tracker might not have to be so reliant on the math. Sometimes A/B/A/B testing is combined with the use of a placebo in a treatment period. Using these methods drawn from science, however, still requires you to make judgments about how long the treatment periods, or exposure periods, should last. Diseases that flare unpredictably, or social expectations, can get in the way of cleanly controlled experiments. An experiment with bedtimes, for example, could be foiled by a spouse's desire to go out dancing.

Cultivating a Habit

Many self-trackers use data to support "habit hacking," or creating new habits and changing old ones. The idea of habit hacking is to change the triggers that create the propensity to do or avoid doing something and create a broader set of routines that support the desired outcome. Habit hackers are attuned to their environment and how it subtly creates cues for practices that one does largely without deliberate thinking. Many take inspiration from the psychologist and persuasive computing innovator B. J. Fogg, who cultivated a flossing habit by starting to floss one tooth only.[19] Easier to do than the whole mouth, and therefore easier to initiate, Fogg's single gesture came to feel over time a part of the "natural" flow of things. He calls this process "tiny habits," where triggering small behaviors can lead to change over time. Self-trackers sometimes talk about "chaining" habits together by timing a new habit like doing sit-ups just after a preexisting habit, like drinking coffee, so that they effectively become one long gesture—a morning routine, say. Psychologists call this "triggering"

Many self-trackers use data to support "habit hacking," or creating new habits and changing old ones.

the behavior, or creating the reminder for an action in the routine.

Habit hacking involves various elements of change—identifying what habits need changing, assessing whether current arrangements in the environment are supporting the ultimate goal, and tinkering with new ways of doing things. Science journalist Charles Duhigg suggests that people ought to focus on changing the "cue" (the circumstances that put someone on autopilot) or "routine" (the set of actions people do to fulfill their underlying desires). He argues that people are less likely to be able to change the underlying "rewards" they seek (relief from boredom, need for social connection, etc.). He suggests replacing the routine with something that brings the same reward in a different way. If a person can identify whether the habit of getting a cookie every afternoon is more about relieving boredom than enjoying the cookie itself, then he can identify a suitable replacement.[20] This is where self-tracking can help. Identifying the cues and routines more clearly can create evidence with which to reflect on what the rewards are really about.

Habit hacking has some constraints. On the one hand, habits are social and contextual, and occur at family, community, and societal levels. A whole family routine cannot be made to change simply because one member needs a new habit. On the other hand, social environments can be arranged to create social "consequences" for an activity. The fear of letting down an exercise partner is a proven way to get more exercise. Self-tracking apps that use motifs and features drawn from games can also motivate by making it clear to others when you did something, even if those others do not actually care if you did it. Whether in social, physical, or virtual environments, habit hacking adjusts environmental and unseen factors in order to change the everyday actions that otherwise easily fall by the wayside.

Practical Considerations for New Habits

Figuring out what triggers an undesired habit, or what the underlying rewards are in a current habit, can help you adapt the techniques of debugging and eliciting sensations. Once you have a clearer sense of what is going on, creating new habits is the next step. B. J. Fogg has a model that follows what is known in psychology: make a goal specific, make it easy to do, and then trigger the behavior. The idea is to map the new habit onto the environment rather than fight against the environment. However, one habit hacker and product manager, who tried an extended form of habit hacking, warned us of just how hard it is to do this. For example, getting to bed earlier might mean rearranging dinnertime, a commute, and childcare, which in turn could impact other elements of the routine. Working with the environment might mean, in practice, inviting more change than you set out to do. Habit hacking could reveal the need for another change, which could prove more problematic than the first. Illness and travel can interfere with a new habit sinking in, and habits take longer to form than most realize. Research shows that twenty-one days might work for simple habits, but "anything harder is likely to take longer to become a really strong habit, and, in the case of some activities, much longer."[21]

There are other self-tracking techniques for supporting the ability to stick with a habit, as opposed to using tracking to understand the nature of the problem. For monitoring a habit that you want to keep, it is often more important to track streaks and consistency. Some have found that representing data in ways that add data cumulatively over a long period of time, rather than relying on daily counts, can be more inspiring. Amelia Greenhall's chart full of shiny gold stars relies on this. Another practice is to use behavioral economics to your own advantage. One app, Beeminder, allows you to place monetary bets on your own success. Complete the practice successfully, and you get your money back. Fail, and the company keeps the money.

What Makes Good Self-Tracking Practice?

Our short foray into various self-tracking techniques makes clear that there is no one way of doing self-tracking right. Some people like Mark Drangsholt take a "science first" approach, where numbers are windows onto an objective truth, and where the role for human bias ought to be minimized. Others, like Robin Barooah or Anne Wright, take a "count first" approach, where the goal might be to reflect on what those perceptions are, or widen one's view of what could be true without worrying about how true it is just yet. The norm within QS is that "good" self-tracking happens when some learning took place, regardless of what kind of learning it was.[22]

Anthropologist Sophie Day and her colleagues have examined the use of numbers outside of science, and pointed out the great many ways that people use numbers. These ways include artistic practices but also a good deal more beyond intellectual reasoning.[23] Numbers are cultural artifacts after all, as human as the art, music, and literature that societies also produce. Even doctors and others who take a "science first" approach do not always use numbers as scientifically accurately as one might think. In a study of statistical literacy among doctors, less than 10 percent correctly solved a word problem asking them to calculate a patient's risk for cancer given information about the probabilities, false positives, and sensitivity of the test.[24] Cross-cultural research shows that people get highly attuned to working with numbers in particular ways, and it can be very difficult to work with them in a style that we are not accustomed to. In a sense, though, no one started out "accustomed to" self-tracking technologies, and in these stories we see evidence of adaptation, and an ability to reconsider previously held views. A scientist expands his view of what counts as evidence while an anthropologist learns to count things without rolling her eyes at the inhumanity of it all. The richness and variety of self-tracking practices that we described here is but a small slice of the diversity of ideas that technology users bring to the table.

In the last sections of this chapter we offer further tips to set up your own self-tracking experiments—tips that are more closely tied to practical concerns. Readers who are not inclined to tinker around with some self-tracking for themselves may simply want to skip ahead to chapter 4 on how the technology industry is shaping self-tracking tools.

Further Practical Considerations

The suggestions that follow are not rules, or canonical best practices, but simply a place to begin if you are curious about starting a project, drawn from our community involvement and in particular Dawn's experience of being coached by Anne Wright. Practices like these do not lend themselves to being codified, and as they pass from person to person, people add their own views or come to modify and adapt them. Undoubtedly, what seems like good advice as we write this might be the worst possible advice for a reader's particular situation. For this reason, we encourage you to start a self-tracking project for a few days and then return to our suggestions, to enlarge the grain of salt with which you will no doubt want to read them.

In terms of getting going, the following are some factors we have learned to consider in gathering self-tracking data.

1. **Start with brevity.** Self-tracking projects should start out as brief experiments that are done, say, over a few days or a few weeks. While there are different benefits to tracking over months or years, a first project should not commit you for the long haul.

2. **Focus on one or two things.** Tracking more than a small number of things makes purposeful attention impossible. Quantification necessarily yields a partial view of daily life, and it is not possible to build a total picture from many partial views. Use partiality to your advantage, as a way to direct your attention to the issues that matter most.

3. **Name those things with care.** Label data in ways that correspond with actual experiences as closely as possible. Questions can sometimes help situate what is being tracked in your actual day-to-day life. For example, tendonitis pain could be tracked with the answers to questions such as "Do you feel up for a hike today?" if being able to hike is what is most relevant to the person who has the tendonitis.

4.   **Time and location are good data curators.** Constraining data collection by time or location can sharpen the point of view your data set provides. Taking a picture once a day at a certain time, or every time you enter a place, is a point of view on your situation. Deciding the time your data records—the overall feeling today, the last few hours, right now—will clarify what it means.

5.   **Be realistic about the work.** Recording something once an hour might work for two days, but for most people that project won't last much longer. Consider how much time and thought you realistically want to give to tracking, and when in the course of the day it is feasible.

6.   **Numbers, words, and pictures all count.** Sometimes jotting down a word or snapping a picture might be the most powerful record of what happened, especially if the time is also automatically recorded. Even the briefest annotations can provide a good record of the context, or help you recall a moment if you need to reconstruct it later. Often sensor data works best in tandem with manually logged notes or other data to make sense of it.

7.   **Numbers have qualities.** If you are using a numerical scale, pay attention to what the scale itself communicates. Scoring things on a five-point scale allows a middle ground; a six-point scale forces you to pick sides. Sometimes a coarser measure—low, medium, or high—is more

effective than having to debate the options of a ten-point scale. You might ask yourself whether a higher or lower number feels more positive or negative to you and assign each end of the scale accordingly. Consider including a number with special meaning as a part of your scale. In statistics the number 9 or 99 often stands in for "missing" data or a question that does not apply. For example, you could track your mood on a scale from 1 to 10, with 99 representing, say, that your mood was not particularly discernable that day.

8. **Words and pictures have quantities.** The frequency of words can be counted so they become number-like. Programs like 750 Words will count keyword frequencies from free text paragraphs, which could provide clues to your preoccupations over time. Some people use 750 Words to track mood by writing a few words every day on the things that made them happy that day. Such programs will also run sentiment analyses to determine whether the tone of the words is positive or negative. Whether you agree with that analysis is another matter.

9. **Self-tracking tools do not have to be fancy.** App developers try to make good guesses about which way of presenting data is likely to be useful, which scales are useful, what words matter, and so on, but these are guesses. Pen and paper logs, Excel, Google Forms, or general-purpose self-reporting apps like Keep Track give you more control

over how things are logged, and more power to change and adapt them as your project changes.

10. **Do a few trial runs.** Chances are pretty good that on your first attempt, something won't be right. Maybe the scale that you've picked for your data might not work well, or the frequency of data collection might be unrealistic. Modifying self-tracking projects before settling on what works is to be expected.

Supposing now that you have done some of these things and have some data in hand, you ask yourself: Now what? Below we list some ways you can analyze data without necessarily embarking on a quest to acquire new statistical or visualization skills. The items in this list are suggestions of how to analyze your data by looking for things that help you spot patterns, find trends, and piece together parts of the puzzle.

1. **Time and location are strong clues.** Most of us naturally look for patterns when we view a graph and try to explain a spike that we see. Often, those patterns indicate something that is not in the data directly—a propensity to visit a restaurant on a certain day of the week, or responsibility for morning childcare duties—that help explain fluctuations in the data. Statisticians often work with time-lagged variables, meaning something produces

an effect later in time. Eating something might trigger a response not immediately but the following day. With time-lagged data, the spikes in the two data sets will not visually line up even if they are related, so you will have to make a temporary adjustment to the time stamp, like adding or subtracting an appropriate amount of hours, before you can see if there is a relationship. Recurrence and time lags can be hard to "eyeball" in a line graph, but there are a few ways of making it more visible. You could print out the graph, and circle each of the "Mondays," for example, to visually amplify the pattern. In a spreadsheet, you could copy the data into a new worksheet, delete all of the data unrelated to the spikes of interest, and then look at the time column to see if there is a time of day or week in common. Visualization software like Data Sense will show recurrences for you automatically, and help you find delayed effects.[25] Fluxtream is a tool optimized for zooming in and out of different time scales, each of which reveals different patterns. If your data has a location stamp, the same principle holds: ask what tends to happen at particular places.

2. **Rolling averages can clarify an underlying trend.** A rolling average shows each data point as an average of the previous few data points. This can be a powerful way to look at data that "smooths" spikes or dips. Weight fluctuates naturally, and a rolling average taken across a week is a better indicator of weight gain or loss than a daily reading

and may create less anxiety. Rolling averages also act as a visual tool when data is dense and has a high amount of variation. When data like this is graphed—imagine calorie data gathered daily over one month—it often looks like many spikes squished together, making the underlying trend hard to see for purely visual reasons. A rolling average can smooth out the variation in the data while preserving the underlying longer-term trend.

3. **Annotate.** Numbers don't tell stories, people do. Jotting down comments onto a chart or inserting pictures can help tell the story in data. If you have been tracking your sleep for a week, and see a dip, you will likely be able to recall the circumstances that led to that dip. If you do this over a few months or a year to try to find the cause of not sleeping well, your recall is less reliable. Anything else you can find—photos, sounds, something you wrote at the time—can help you draw connections between what you are tracking and what you didn't track.

4. **Collages support visual sensemaking.** When photos of the same thing (food, pills, faces) are shown in a series, patterns can emerge through shape and color. Tracking in this way makes mathematical calculations more difficult, but visual patterns can yield more viscerally powerful feedback than numbers.[26] Things inadvertently captured about the location, or the packaging of an object, or other people accidentally caught in the shot, can also help you recall the

context, or capture additional information that you might not have thought to include at first.

5.   **Missing data isn't really absent.** Patches of missing data have meaning. They could mean that things have gone in an embarrassing or troubling direction, making it more emotionally difficult to record data, or that the issue has resolved itself. If you have a theory about whether your missing data is likely to have been lower or higher than the overall average, you can mentally revise up or down any averages or correlations that have been calculated. Missing data can also *become* data itself. If you are tracking a particular activity, looking at the patterns of *not* doing something might lead you to different explanations than if you look at what *was* done.

6.   **Telling the story is an opportunity to craft it.** There is an open secret of QS show-and-tell talks. People take the time to think more carefully about their data when they have to explain it to someone else. That is when the full story of their data emerges. Talking through your data with someone else and discovering what others see in it can be another useful mirror alongside the data itself.

7.   **Comparisons with other people can provide context.** Most self-trackers we talk to do not find it helpful to ask whether their data deviates from the average across a population. Seeing examples of other people's data, however,

gives a view into possible variation. We saw, for example, one Portland self-tracker complaining that a sleep-quality algorithm must not be very good, because he found it impossible to get a score below 95 percent. Another chimed in, saying he had used the same device, and indeed a low score is possible, which gave the first self-tracker insight into his own data.

Once you have had the opportunity to look at your data, some of you will likely look for changes to make. Obviously, we cannot tell you what to do, but there are some resources worth considering if you get stuck. Nutritionists, naturopaths, mental health professionals, and others who take holistic approaches are often more interested in self-tracking data than overworked doctors, who, for reasons we go into in chapter 5, often would rather not see self-tracking data. There is also a nascent field of *data coaches* who are not medically trained, but understand self-tracking techniques well and might have some experience with the problem at hand. A good data coach will let you lead, such that you are still *self*-tracking, just with more resources and feedback at your disposal.

Disease-specific online communities can have very knowledgeable participants with extensive first-hand experience, and often people talk about their data on forums. If you have data in hand, communities like Patients Like Me or Cure Together can be an excellent place to talk about both data and experiences. If you live in an urban area, your local Quantified Self meetup group will be a welcoming place to ask questions and solicit advice. We also list some additional resources in the back of this book.

Collecting data creates a perceived burden to respond in some way.[27] If you have tracked caffeine hoping it could alleviate symptoms, and it emerges that how much caffeine you drink does not really matter, you could find that your tracking practice created a false sense of control, and ultimately disappointment. Experiments can and do fail, and choosing what you do *not* want to know is as important as choosing what to know. Still, it is worth remembering that one successful resolution to a problem is to decide that it is not, in fact, a problem. We have seen plenty of examples of people using data to quiet their worries. The same person who tracked glucose in the story in this chapter also tracked his mood and his sleep, though for different reasons. When he put the mood and sleep data sets together, he found that the days he was in a foul mood were often days when he had poor sleep the night before. His potential problem thus became a nonproblem—a reversal of the more common commercial practice of using quantification to create and legitimize "problems" we did not know we had.

Now that we've looked at the communities and the practices of self-tracking, we turn in chapter 4 to the tools and devices—and the industries that are producing them.

SELF-TRACKING AND THE TECHNOLOGY INDUSTRY

The invitation was simple enough: meet for a coffee in the coolest café in a neighborhood known for its density of tech company headquarters. Gina had met someone at a health innovation conference who had experience in luxury consumer goods and left to work on a self-tracking device. But at this follow-up meeting, it was not the ethnographer asking the questions. Hanging in the air was the question that neither Gina nor a whole host of technology companies could yet answer: "What are we going to do with all this data?"

"What are we going to do with all this data?" is an important question. The data from self-tracking tools enjoys none of the privacy and security protections that are required of health data, and yet it often paints just as intimate a picture of our lives. Exactly how much of people's data is also used for marketing, whether its use has discriminatory effects, or whether it reduces costs to provide a service are all important to know. Self-tracking data is already being used to differentiate among customers in marketing, but it could cross a line into discrimination if it is used as a proxy for gender, race, or religion. As money is made from data, companies' abilities to track you might be more financially valuable to them than supporting your capacity to keep track of yourself. Indeed, there are parts of the private sector where self-tracking might be more accurately called "self"-tracking, because it is not really by or for the self at all.

That people in the private sector are still asking, "What are we going to do with all this data?" implies attitudes towards self-tracking data that should concern everyone. As self-tracking tools go mainstream, they are developed and defined, at least initially, in terms set by a large and complex industry. That industry gives the rest of us a set of social operating instructions—initial communications about what new devices do, who they are for, and how they should be used. When industry actors say, "What are we going to do with all this data?" they imply that at some level, the companies themselves do not yet know who or what self-tracking devices are for. It is a question rife with ambiguity, unusual for an industry that generally does not tolerate unclear claims about return on investment. It is an industry that values, as critic Evgeny Morozov puts it, "efficiency, transparency, certitude, and perfection."[1] Why, then, do so many business models for self-tracking tools hinge on such vagueness?

The answer has to do with the cultural norms that the technology industry works under and a lack of clarity surrounding regulatory scrutiny. These two factors shape how markets develop, leaving consumers with unclear or underwhelming messages about what their data can do for them. The technology industry currently has a good deal of control over who gets tools designed for them, and what kinds of values those tools reflect or reproduce in the world, which is a good reason to examine some of the more common industrial practices.

What We Mean by "the Industry"

The interests of people who work in technology are not unified and coherent. Self-tracking tools are sometimes developed by individuals, activists, and patient groups far from Silicon Valley. In many cases, they are developed within universities and then commercialized. As the wearables and digital health markets have matured, however, self-tracking technologies have gained enormous attention and funding from powerful interests. Over forty-two million fitness trackers a year will be sold by 2019.[2] While official data was not yet available when we wrote this, one analyst estimated that seven million Apple Watches were sold in the product's first six months.[3] Across Silicon Valley, venture capital funding for digital health has grown explosively. In 2014 funding for digital health companies exceeded $4.1 billion, a total almost greater than that of the prior three years combined. This funding is coming from established venture capital firms like Sequoia, Andreessen Horowitz, Kleiner Perkins Caufield Byers, and Khosla Ventures, as well as from corporate investments made by Merck, Google, Qualcomm, and Cambia, a health insurance company. Digital health funding is growing at a faster rate than venture capital funding in general. The top areas for funding within digital health are analytics and big data, healthcare consumer engagement, digital medical devices, telemedicine, personalized medicine, and population health management.[4] Many of these areas concern producing self-tracking tools, or use data from those tools in some way.

This influx of money has meant that the ecology of the self-tracking industry now includes traditional technology giants, massive medical device companies, pharmaceutical companies, insurance companies, large hospital groups, and sportswear companies and luxury brands. These different kinds of companies have different agendas for wearable technologies and their associated data. Individual creators and "makers" still play a role, however. Quantified Self meetups are full of people who have day jobs designing and making self-tracking technologies, but put on new hats as technology users, advocates, "hackers" (people who adapt technologies for a new purpose), or hobbyist inventors. These multiple roles give people a way to reflect on what they do in their day job.[5] Dawn is no stranger to this, as someone who works for a large technology firm while also participating in the debates about data access, and product usefulness within QS. She designs research at Intel in different ways and suggests different technical directions, as a result of her interpersonal exchanges. Even though the boundary between the categories of *technology makers* and *users* is sometimes blurred, the two are useful in examining how industrial processes help to define the initial social operating instructions of new devices and tools, and how and when these definitions diverge from how people use them in practice.

How Industrial Actors See Their Markets

Several factors contribute to what industry actors see in self-tracking devices and data, and why there is so much market enthusiasm. The first is that the technology has matured. Sensor systems can now be used reliably, and be produced at a price that some people can pay. Innovations including the rise of smartphones, Bluetooth, GPS, and accelerometers have led to new "form factors," an industry term for the material envelopes for the technology inside. Technological innovations make smaller devices conceivable, but it is the social and material envelopes for them that help us imagine wearing them on our bodies. For instance, the social practices behind a smartwatch are older than the technology, such as the tradition of people wearing a wristwatch as status jewelry. While these technologies are now in play, their relative newness contributes to the mysterious quality of "what we will do with all this data." The tools are indeed at the edge of social change; we learn over time how to make sense of the numbers they yield by trying them out in real-world situations.

The second factor behind such high levels of investment is the social changes we've already outlined that make tracking oneself appealing, including biomedicalization and the turn to a data-centric culture more generally. Biomedicalization has affected the technology industry somewhat differently than it has affected the general public. Pointing to medical expertise while proposing a business plan creates a sense of certainty that the plan could work. It gives the plan an aura of authority, especially when controversies in science are downplayed. In fact, a recent study compared the analysis of the metaphors used in a wearables trade show and Body Worlds, the science museum show that displays dead bodies encased in plastic.[6] The language and metaphors were nearly indistinguishable, showing just how much confidence wearables manufacturers have that we already know what we are looking at when we look at data. To them, the data is as self-evident in its representation of bodies as a muscle or a tendon in an anatomic dissection. This confidence comes at a cost. Companies are less likely to design for the potentially valuable knowledge that might emerge in the course of using data, and finding out what it really means in practice. This is knowledge that might not yet be acknowledged by medical or aligned fields.

Both biomedicine and businesses see things through the lens of probabilities. These probabilities, like "women who exercise are likely to be less stressed," hold true across a population, or a market. Generic probabilities offer a degree of certainty that customers will respond in a certain way—a certainty that businesses crave. Probabilities "tame chance," as historian Ian Hacking would say, and when chance is tamed, investment can flow.[7] When industry actors hear phrases like "women who exercise are likely to be less stressed," it is a short leap to try to codify it into data form, and design, say, a technology that recommends more exercise to reduce stress. This leads companies to optimize their designs for the overall probability and to treat other factors within the individual context of use as "noise," too hard to account for in the design, or defend as a good way to spend resources. That "noise" of personal context, though, makes or breaks technology adoption, so businesses ignore it at their peril.

This leads us to our third factor. Companies very much want to believe that their technologies are good at solving problems. Evgeny Morozov has called this faith "technological solutionism," the idea that complex social problems can be solved by technology alone.[8] Technological solutionism elevates technology companies to a privileged role in solving complex problems and downplays roles that others could play. We can see solutionism at work in the provocative language of a *Time* magazine article reporting on Google's new long-term health project, titled "Google vs. Death."[9] Excesses like these are clearly absurd, yet individual careers are often rewarded for indulging in them. However, our own experience in industry leads us to believe that frequently there is also something more modest at work—a human desire for building something that matters to others. Nevertheless, this tendency toward solutionism dissuades firms from closely examining whether data is actually a good or appropriate solution to a proposed problem. Solutionism says technologies impact people and not the other way around, so firms are less inclined to spend the resources necessary to understand the social dynamics their products depend on to have an effect. This is a particularly risky strategy for data products, as the meaning of data is directly tied to these dynamics. Investment dollars may follow grand claims untouched by social reality, but many self-tracking tools flounder because they are not clearly tied to existing practices or communities where people can make sense of their data.

Finally, the fourth factor generating commercial interest in self-tracking data is its potential for centralization.

In Silicon Valley, data is seen as a valuable general-purpose resource to stockpile—"the new oil" that might one day serve multiple, potential purposes. A common idea within Silicon Valley is that businesses are really about "democratization" or "horizontalization." For example, distributed networks like the Internet have in some senses distributed access to the means of communication more widely. However, the industry is also intensely preoccupied with the question of which company will become the next "platform"—the next hub into which all the other elements in the system must connect, and where the platform owner can start to extract money from the other actors in that system. Many of the famous Silicon Valley firms have made money by putting themselves at the center of a distributed network of some kind—whether sellers and buyers in the case of Amazon, or friends and acquaintances in the case of Facebook. There is much start-up activity where firms attempt to become a central hub for self-tracking data.

The interest in centralization in an otherwise distributed system means that there is tremendous pressure for business plans to "scale," that is, attract many customers or partners. When new product developers propose a plan, they have a "use case," that describes what they believe people will do with their product. Artificially tidy use cases, like "people want to be able to monitor their health" shuffle away the mess of real life, and make "scale" more conceivable.[10] After all, who *wouldn't* want to monitor their

In Silicon Valley, data is seen as a valuable general-purpose resource to stockpile—"the new oil" that might one day serve multiple, potential purposes.

health? Most anthropologists who work in industry regularly see how hard it is for companies to fully embrace the realities of what people actually do, because those messy realities make some business practices harder. Messy reality makes it harder to imagine how a product could "scale up," because each context has its own set of confounding factors. It is easier for product managers to work with generic statements that can be put into a survey, which can then be can be statistically inferred to make claims about a larger market, even though those statements might not be meaningful to anyone in particular. Data products are no exception. It is hard for industrial actors to hear the voices of independent self-trackers describing what truly suits them. Reality, however, does eventually catch up. When business people finally do jump into the mess of handling data, they can be surprised that they then must ask themselves, "What are we going to do with all this data?"

The Economic Role of Data

Given these ways that industry actors approach data, the question then becomes: How is money currently being made, and do these ways of making money have social effects that we need to consider? Here we will focus on the consumer market. In general, there are a few different ways that data is used in economic activity. First, many firms gather data that they believe might be directly useful to customers. The self-tracking data *is* the product, as with heart rate monitors, run trackers, and direct-to-consumer blood sample analysis. Second, firms gather data that may enhance their service relationship with customers. For example, the apps Runtastic and Runkeeper provide additional personalized coaching for a premium, and the ability to personalize the coaching service relies on data. Nest, the Internet-enabled thermostat company, has announced they have entered into relationships with utilities firms in order to offer services that balance energy consumption across the grid.[11] The ability to balance energy use across the grid relies on the exchange of data between the two kinds of firms. Third, companies that rely on advertising for their revenue generally use data to determine where and to whom to target those advertisements and other kinds of marketing. This is a widespread way of doing business that is not limited to self-tracking. Some firms make money by analyzing overall patterns in the data sets they assemble. For example, the genetics testing company 23andMe entered a $60 million deal to give the biotech company Genentech (a subsidiary of global pharmaceutical giant Roche) access to the data from 23andMe customers.[12]

In chapter 3 we showed how many people were in fact getting valuable information from self-tracking devices. Here we must also acknowledge that the data generated in these devices is a part of a broader economy in which data plays a role. Do these various ways of making money from data disadvantage customers in some way? Whether an exchange is fair or not may have more to do with the particular circumstances than whether a firm makes any money or what the particular parties consider fair. The specifics are important.

For example, some companies consider self-tracking data to be the property of their customers, while other companies consider such data to be theirs. The patterns in the "population level" data—that is, data that has been analyzed by the company and stripped of information that makes it easy to identify individuals—might have a different set of ownership rights associated with it than the raw data. Terms of Service documents are notoriously difficult to read, widely ignored, and at times so broadly written that they say very little about what companies actually do with their users' data. However, some companies also offer a version with less legal jargon or make some other attempts to communicate what is happening with customers' data. Some companies are very strict about ensuring all activities that concern people's data happen on an opt-in basis, while other companies offer the ability to opt-out if they believe that there is little risk to the person, and that an opt-in policy would make providing an otherwise valuable service impossible. These are important variations in what firms do, and are the kinds of practices worth examining before becoming a customer of any particular company.

While there are meaningful differences between various business practices, legal scholar Frank Pasquale has argued that companies that handle data have, in general, become less transparent rather than more.[13] A lack of transparency in what is going to happen on the basis of data makes it difficult for people to make meaningful choices about what they are willing to opt into. Pasquale calls this the "black box society," referring both to the digital "black boxes" similar to those on airplanes that provide increasingly detailed views of people's lives, and to "black boxes" in the engineering sense—systems where we do not understand the inner workings but we nevertheless use them.

The area of greatest concern in the black box society is the secondary use of data. Pasquale cites the case of a couple using a credit card to access mental health services, only to find that their credit score was negatively impacted as a result. They were judged to be risky people to offer credit to, not people who were seeking to solve an unrelated problem. While not every instance of data collection leads to a situation as serious as this, Pasquale's point is that the potential for issues of this magnitude to arise is very real. He argues that the creation of data, or the handling of data in the private sector is not, inherently, a bad thing. In fact, his book offers potential remedies to improve the situation based on his expertise in law and political economy. He is not the only one looking for ways to improve this situation. The White House convened a

Big Data and Privacy Working Group in 2014 to identify ways to address the social issues raised by widespread use of big data, while retaining data's practical and economic value.[14] Engineers who work on machine learning (the techniques used to find patterns in large data sets) are also asking questions about how to design algorithms in ways that avoid harmful biases, and how to design algorithms with a greater sensitivity toward the potential social consequences of the results.[15]

Making Markets in Self-Tracking

Making a market for self-tracking tools involves defining the products being sold and communicating how they should be used. Right now, self-tracking tools are in several markets. Yet, the technology industry still struggles to find compelling definitions for the tools being released. According to a report from Rock Health, a company that supports startups and tracks investments in digital health, most connected sensing devices lack clear definitions: "The generic marketing language of most devices leaves use cases to the purchaser's imagination."[16] The reasons we offered earlier— technological newness, an inflated sense of data's certainty, the perceived need to stay generic in order to scale, and, of course, solutionism—show why such generic language is common for the marketing of self-tracking tools.

Key areas are already beginning to cohere. One market area involves designing self-tracking tools as luxury items sold alongside high-end jewelry and accessories. Fashion designer Tory Burch designed a set of luxury jewelry accessories for Fitbit, fashion CEO Angela Ahrendts left Burberry to help Apple with launching the Apple Watch, Swiss watchmaker Tag Heuer collaborated with Google and Intel on a smartwatch, the fashion company Rebecca Minkoff has designed smart devices into its accessories line, and activity tracker Misfit designed a device built into a Swarovski crystal. Another direction involves building sports performance devices that professional athletes help to sell to an army of weekend warriors looking to improve their performance on ten-kilometer runs or triathlons or Cross-Fit workouts. Professional triathlete Timothy O'Donnell helps to market Garmin's smartwatches with the image that these tools are for serious athletic uses. Meanwhile, professional sports teams are equipping players with biometric trackers from STAT Sports, Zephyr, and Catapult sports, while amateurs are flocking to fitness studios like Orangetheory Fitness that use the public display of heart rate monitoring as part of group training sessions.[17] Yet another market area for self-tracking treats tools as communication lifelines between doctors and their patients, serving to help inform decisions, enable elders' independence, or incentivize healthier activities. French medical device company Withings suggests that doctors in Europe and the United States should be prescribing their at-home blood pressure cuffs and scales to better coordinate care. If so, then self-tracking tools are suited for use in medical contexts, which the technology industry has been slow to tackle and medical device makers have been slow to add on. Finally, a substantial market has emerged in workplace monitoring, where employers are sold devices that track employees in various ways, sometimes to keep track of the jobs they do, and at other times to keep track of their non-work activities as a way to keep healthcare provision costs down. Gartner research says that ten thousand companies worldwide offered their employees fitness trackers and that as of 2016 most companies with more than five hundred employees will offer them.[18] These emerging markets reveal which kinds of problems the industry believes it can solve through a consumer market. They also shape who has access to these tools and in what circumstances.

Self-tracking tools are emerging at the intersections of key social arenas—between health and wellness, between work and life, and between accessibility and luxury. These intersections further muddy the social operating instructions that device manufacturers might have otherwise communicated. For example, medical uses for fitness tracking devices and platforms can't be encouraged or commented upon by the companies making a market in consumer wellness. People managing their diabetes might use, say, Jawbone UP and its data platform and the

Self-tracking tools
are emerging at the
intersections of key
social arenas—between
health and wellness,
between work and
life, and between
accessibility and luxury.

company's carbohydrate counter. But if the company were to publically encourage the use of the device for managing diabetes it could run afoul of regulators. Similarly, devices are accessible in the sense that they can be cheaper than professional healthcare services and tools, but the luxury product lines and adoption patterns that create cultural associations between these new technologies and the young, healthy, and rich make them less accessible socially. To further explain what we mean, we look closer at three of these emerging markets—what we will call the health line, the luxury line, and the work line.

The Health Line

At least in the United States, healthism informs consumer markets. Look no further than the shelves of a Whole Foods supermarket to see the blurred line between "health" as a kind of consumer activity and set of identities, and something that could be called "healthcare." It is an enormous gray zone comprised of aisles of supplements, food fads, health trends, and diet choices that reside somewhere between a medical recommendation and cultural desire to consume one's way to health. On this shelf we find ideas about "healthy living" that are based on popular interpretations of medical and quasi-medical knowledge. "Healthy living" in the context of a consumer market is different from healthcare in fundamental ways, but this does not stop companies from making use of popular notions of health that muddy the distinction. Whether or not people should be looking to the technology industry to help solve health problems is yet another consideration.

Self-tracking tools are designed for consumers who are young and already fit. This raises concerns. Companies encourage some people to consume their way to "health," while ignoring other, potentially less profitable, customers. Marketing materials for activity trackers show extreme bodies that fit a narrow image of what healthy looks like, by showing people who are young and fit using these devices. But look at what happens when companies venture outside this presumption. We quickly find ourselves in a different market, the "independent living" market, one where older people are treated as if they are only ever in need of surveillance, where other human needs like beauty or curiosity somehow just disappear.

The independent living market is an active one. According to a 2014 survey, two of every three seniors want to use self-care technology to independently manage their health, and 62 percent are willing to wear a health-monitoring device to track vital signs.[19] Lively is one product designed specifically for seniors that combines the same sort of activity tracking we see in the fitness market with sensors around the home to help monitor if a person is taking her medicines on schedule, how frequently she goes outside, and how often she opens the refrigerator, to monitor for signs of confusion or distress. In some situations, such sensors may enable seniors to live independently for longer. Some studies, though, indicate that many people would rather not live under the scrutiny involved in using such systems. Regardless of whether independent living products are designed wisely, what is left on the table in the "health line" are people who do not fit the mold of the young body that can be optimized, or the mold of the docile body in need of extensive management by others. The industry has little to say to those in between—the injured, the disabled, the poor, or the middle-aged—unless they too share the same narrow view of what an optimal body is.

The Luxury Line

Self-tracking tools also sit at an intersection of luxury accessory and mass-market consumer items. From the Apple Watch to the designer cuff, many self-tracking consumer devices attempt to appeal as luxury goods. They are designed to help relatively wealthy people have more fashionable bodies, flaunt a technology insider's knowledge, or show the world a status symbol. These markets work because exclusivity is balanced with a large enough customer base for profitability. Luxury marketing communicates the idea that self-tracking tools are optional, exclusive, and about the presentation of personal style to others who also value conspicuous consumption. Luxury goods also handle potentially medically useful data sets. The promise of Apple's HealthKit, the development package for creating apps compliant with HIPAA (the Health Insurance Portability and Accountability Act), the regulation that governs US healthcare data, is that it allows one device to link social uses with health uses with fashionable ones.

Again, we see a market being made at social intersections, where the industry wrestles with how to handle social distinctions like class. For the wealthy, what appears as a choice to wear this or that consumer product might feel like necessity—a pressure to be seen to be consuming in the right way. How will tracking technologies intersect with what one sociologist calls the "glamour labor" needed to make and maintain fashionable bodies? Indeed, the work involved might be quite real for many. "Huge sections of the populace don activity trackers . . . download health-enhancement apps, track their sleep habits, and log their nutrition practices and goals, ostensibly in pursuit of the body beautiful, while blogging, Facebooking, and tweeting about their accomplishments and watching their Klout scores all the while."[20] Just reading the list can be exhausting enough. Fashionable luxury tools may further set up unattainable measures for bodies—an unattainability that has historically affected women more seriously, but might affect men in new ways, too.

The "healthy lifestyle" that is sold with the Apple Watch is only available for those who can afford to buy it. According to Carl Cederström and André Spicer, conspicuous wellness, or what they call the "wellness syndrome," casts a new light on people who cannot afford to consume their way to wellness, or who otherwise do not buy into it. They argue that society increasingly sees them as a kind of weak-willed degenerate class in a social system already too prepared to see poor people as lazy. They write, "Where does our preoccupation with our own wellness leave the rest of the population, who have an acute shortage of organic smoothies, diet apps and yoga instructors?"[21] Most connected wearable devices already on the market, even those outside the luxury line, come with the presumption that their owners also have both a smartphone and a computer, which is not necessarily the case for the elderly, poor, and sick. Forty percent of adults in the United States report that they foresee buying some kind of wearable device. This indicates that wearables extend well beyond a luxury market, but luxury marketing sends signals about which wearable technologies are "for" the mass market, creating class and identity distinctions among self-tracking tools.

One writer points out the conundrum this situation poses for many people: even if we "are not all thoroughly brainwashed by the wellness syndrome, it is still universal to find oneself seduced by some aspect [of it] . . . say, wanting to get better at one thing or another."[22] There is nothing inherently snobbish, elite or misguided about wanting to see whether doing something differently could make you happier. It does not make you a sheepish consumer to look for the most readily available tools to do it. However, when wellness becomes shorthand for all these class identities and is used to make distinctions between luxury and mass markets, we must acknowledge that this poses problems for social inclusion. Companies use a sort of social shorthand to communicate what their products do, and they pick up on the most readily available concept, one they think most people will recognize. Mobilizing concepts of "wellness" in this way might not ultimately serve the industry well in the long run. Such marketing excludes many kinds of people, encourages the abandonment of design directions that do not fit the cultural politics but could be viable for other reasons, and invites rejection from people turned off by those particular images of wellness.

The Work Line

Factories perhaps were the first place where people's activities were quantified at scale, with workers clocking in and out and management practices that measured minute details of time and motion in an attempt to optimize the productivity of workers' every gesture. Companies already use wearables like wristbands and headbands to monitor the productivity of warehouse workers in real time and GPS to track truck and delivery drivers for improved "logistics" productivity.[23] Office workers are highly tracked through productivity software that, in the words of one writer, can "drill down and micromanage the work of their single employees or teams of employees."[24]

Now, companies are using self-tracking tools to encourage healthier lifestyles among their employees, which companies see as lowering their health insurance costs or increasing workers' productivity in a different way. Industry analyst group ABI Research predicts that 13 million wearable activity trackers will be deployed or subsidized as part of corporate wellness programs.[25] The American Heart Association claims that for every dollar spent on corporate wellness programs, the company saves three, while *Harvard Business Review* cites studies that paint a more mixed economic picture.[26]

As with the other lines, we see the same familiar social intersections at play. Changes in contemporary office work have blurred the line between home and work, and employees are expected to care passionately about their work regardless of where they are. Wearables acquired through work change what nonwork time is for. They make nonwork time increasingly about creating a rested, strong body capable of more work and make it harder for people to also care for family members, for example, or pursue civic or artistic activities. With some exceptions, companies are generally not offering reduced workloads to make room for more exercise and sleep. If fifty-, sixty-, and seventy-hour workweeks are still required, something must give. Flexible work hours do not solve the fundamental problem that there are only twenty-four hours in a day. We would not be surprised to see employees questioning why these benefits to firms must come at the expense of childcare, eldercare, and other equally important matters.

We also see class playing a role here. Warehouse workers do not have a problem with being sedentary, and "their" tracking data is really about the company managing an industrial process. Office workers have at least a chance that the employer will not see the data. The handling of data brings us straight to the intersection with medical practice, because part of employers' incentive is to reduce healthcare premiums. Whether health insurance companies have access to employee data—and if they do, whether it is at the individual level or aggregated across the employee base—varies by company. Regardless of where the data goes, the obligation to create a body that is perceived as productive and worthy is a real pressure. One workplace study of employee activity tracking found that the firm's "step challenge" created a divide among employees, and even participants were immensely relieved when it was over. Another study showed that otherwise happy employees, become anxious about losing their jobs after the introduction of a corporate wellness program. They worry about their employability, knowing they will be expected to measure up and achieve various "wellness" benchmarks that might not be possible for them. A University of Pennsylvania experiment showed that these workplace wellness programs might not help people lose weight even when there are financial incentives of more than $500 involved.[27] Employers' willingness to invest in the physical well-being of their employees must be recognized as a good thing on the whole, but we see little evidence that care is being taken to ensure their investments do not have perverse effects.

The Regulatory Patchwork

These social intersections create confusion about which regulations apply where. A consumer device subsidized by an employer may or may not fall under the jurisdiction of labor law. Foods, supplements, and tools are regularly sold as part of a "healthy lifestyle" but there comes a point where the regulation of medicine does in fact kick in. In the United States, regulation is fragmented across different kinds of agencies and different sets of rules. For example, the Federal Trade Commission (FTC) regulates safety of consumer products, and is active in ensuring data security, though some companies have challenged whether they have the right to do so. The Federal Communications Commission (FCC) also plays a role, especially where telecommunications firms are involved. The Food and Drug

Administration (FDA) decides what is and is not a medical device, while Health and Human Services (HHS) enforces the health data privacy legislation HIPAA. These regulations are regularly tested in courts and can shift in practice.

So how is privacy regulated and enforced? Unlike the European Union, the United States has no omnibus privacy legislation, which means the federal government has effectively chosen not to set overall norms with respect to privacy. Some legislation, such as the Americans with Disabilities Act, Genetic Information Non-Discrimination Act, and the entirely voluntary Fair Information Practice Principles (FIPPs) provide some guidance for how companies should protect privacy in some circumstances. Some states offer some protections for employees' rights to engage in lawful activities outside of work without risk of job termination, but employers can easily circumvent these laws by requiring employees to sign contracts "agreeing" to employer surveillance over their nonwork activities, and accepting termination if they run afoul of employer rules. HIPAA applies only when data is collected in a medical setting. Blood pressure data collected in a clinical setting enjoys HIPAA protections, while blood pressure data collected by a consumer device at home does not. Whether it is "more private" in one space or the other is debatable, and companies might choose to make their apps HIPAA-compliant if it enables integration with medical practice.

Because data is social—it goes places, and aggregates in various ways—this patchwork regulatory landscape can become a problem for companies. The practical reality is that people with chronic conditions turn to off-the-shelf wellness tools to help manage their conditions. A person with diabetes might use a general dieting app to help track carbs to help her calibrate her insulin intake, and it could be better to have companies acknowledge it rather than ignore it. Others may want to modify that same tool to help them detect subtle changes in their condition over time, and find they suddenly have a "medical device" on their hands that they can legally use themselves, but not share with others. Other people still may post their health and wellness data on social media and patient forums, thus making the forum owner suddenly an inadvertent handler of medical data. Companies have struggled to figure out how to keep open the possibilities of users getting the most out of their tools without suggesting uses that might not be approved by regulators. There are now FDA guidelines about what constitutes a mobile medical device and more precedents now compared to the emergence of the consumer market for self-tracking. These help provide examples of the kinds of practices that may run afoul of regulations. New sorts of questions, of course, will always arise as new technologies come to the market.

This difficult patchwork, on top of the many other reasons we identified, is an important reason that companies' messages about their products are so generic and uninformative. They generally leave it to others to do the work of figuring out what data could mean for problems that people truly find pressing, like what triggers their migraines or what could be done to relieve their exhaustion. That is yet another form of labor that consumers are left to do on their own, unpaid, either in web forums or through voluntary groups and organizations. They might even have to pay a data coach to do it. Often companies host web forums to help their customers talk about product-related issues, but it is the consumers doing the work of figuring it out. Creating spaces for sharing—data, ideas, tips, values—in such forums requires careful balancing of the interests of the commercial enterprise and community-driven values, and these may or may not align in the brand/product online communities set up by technology companies.

The bigger barrier to making markets, in our view, lies in how companies' own business processes sanitize and genericize, making many firms unable to appreciate just how much self-tracking data could matter to people. As these markets mature, generic "wellness" and "fitness" will no longer do. The usefulness of data products, more than other kinds of products, is highly context-specific. The companies that can truly embrace the mess and noise of how data is really used in everyday life will fare far better in the long run even if, in the short run, these things are difficult to talk about in the next pitch meeting.

In the next chapter, we turn to how self-tracking tools are being used within medicine.

SELF-TRACKING AND MEDICINE

An important hope for self-tracking is that it can improve people's health and wellness, and this hope plays a large role in the rhetoric of healthcare technology innovators. The daily tracking of symptoms, metrics, and outcomes has long been a part of the home care for people managing chronic conditions. All new mothers are asked to track their babies' "output" as a proxy for how well the babies are feeding. For clinics, tracking is not new.

Medicine raises just as many social questions as the consumer market in self-tracking. Here too, our own data can be used against us. It can be used by others like insurance companies to manage our health through incentives, punishments, or rewards that exert tight control over our daily activities. Controlling our health in this way requires knowing what "normal" and "healthy" actually *are* for a population, and yet the more extensively we measure ourselves, the more extensively that knowledge is being challenged. Strong social, cultural, and economic forces may nevertheless marshal that data for control and profit, especially where there are economic incentives to do so.

Self-tracking presents enormous challenges to regulated systems of clinical care. Public health advocates hope self-tracking tools can help people change unhealthy habits. This prospect can become reality only if tools and apps are designed with realistic behavior-change models in mind, if their differing goals for tracking are met, and if people are in control of their data. Unfortunately, these three conditions are not widespread yet. Some believe self-tracking will bring down the cost of healthcare and therefore improve access to healthcare in parts of the world where costs have skyrocketed, like the United States, or never have been accessible by the majority, as is the case in large parts of the developing world. Innovations that use smartphones to put portable and cheap devices in the hands of many people outside the clinic have the potential to both bring down costs and improve access, but this will not happen without social innovation as well. Meanwhile, doctors worry about what new kinds of data might mean for their workload in their already overloaded practices. While many self-tracking projects never actually involve doctors, this chapter focuses on how healthcare providers encounter self-tracking tools and practices and the political and economic forces that could turn an individual's data into either a tool for improving their health or for discriminating against them.

Self-tracking to monitor and improve health has already become a common practice. According to a 2013 Pew Research Center Internet & American Life Project survey report, 69 percent of Americans keep track of some kind of health data for themselves or a loved one—47 percent do so "in their heads," while the rest either keep track with pen and paper (33 percent) or a digital technology (20 percent).[1] People with serious chronic conditions are more likely to track and are more likely to do so using a medical device. Sixty-two percent of Americans with two or more chronic conditions report tracking, which suggests that some people with chronic conditions may already use their self-tracking data in conversations with their healthcare providers. Most self-trackers responded that tracking led them to changes in their approach to their health, new questions of their doctors, and different health decisions. Still, half of all US health trackers update their information "only occasionally at most" and do not share their information with anyone else. Of those who do share, 52 percent of them share with their doctors or care providers.[2] Our question is not whether self-tracking data will be used in clinical healthcare settings, but rather *how* and under what terms. A conversation with a doctor about a blood pressure reading at home has different implications than that same reading being integrated into an electronic health record. This data matters for health, whether the impetus for tracking comes from a healthcare provider, a technology maker, a DIY enthusiast, or oneself. Self-tracking and DIY enthusiasts can step in where formal healthcare systems have left gaps, but once self-tracking encounters clinical practices additional social forces shape the data and what happens to it.

Empowering Patients

An example of what patient empowerment through self-tracking might look like is the Nightscout project. Started by parents of children with Type 1 Diabetes, Nightscout is an open-source, do-it-yourself modification of a continuous blood glucose monitor that displays the monitor's data onto a smartwatch or smartphone. There are many situations where someone might want to do this. With Nightscout, a parent could monitor glucose levels of his child who is away at a sleepover. An adult can reduce the disruption to her social life caused by constantly having to look at a glucose monitor that others believe to be a "pager," and is freed from needing to interact with the "pager" while doing a two-handed activity. And Nightscout's flexibility means she can glance at her blood glucose on a watch rather than a smartphone while driving. Changing how and where data is displayed helps enormously for managing the disease.

Nightscout encapsulates many of the issues that emerge when self-tracking meets medicine. Nightscout shows what kinds of innovation are possible from users, patients, and their loved ones. It also shows some of the complications that arise from the distinction between clinical and nonclinical data. For example, Nightscout changes which screen the data is displayed on—from a single purpose monitor display, to a display that the user is more likely to see. It does not recalculate that data, or make a medical recommendation, but the US Food and Drug Administration (FDA) asserts the rights over medical device data displayed in different formats. Regulators want to be sure that readings are not lost in the translation and that they are safe and reliable. However, the designers behind the Nightscout project, and the people who have joined in, have organized through the Twitter campaign #WeAreNotWaiting. They say they are not waiting either for regulatory approval or for device makers to design a solution. As they put it, #WeAreNotWaiting "for others to decide if, when, and how we access and use data from our own bodies."[3] While they are unable to exchange the technology on the marketplace, the project teaches parents and patients how to deploy the open source software on their own to get it working with their devices.[4]

While Nightscout takes a do-it-yourself approach, others have different ideas about what empowerment might look like. Some companies are looking to passive monitoring to help with challenges in medication adherence, and the pharmaceutical industry is exceedingly interested in tools that help ensure that people continue taking (and buying) their pharmaceuticals. They claim that patients are empowered by being able to take their medicines at home rather than having to go to the doctor's office or be overseen by another healthcare provider. While this claim has serious social implications that we discuss in this chapter, it shows how information technologies blur the boundaries between clinic and home care. Smartphones and other devices change where healthcare happens.

Self-tracking data may also change the power relationships within medicine. Patients, clinicians, and medical researchers have to renegotiate roles for data in healthcare and disease management. Healthcare professionals still must figure out how to evaluate patient self-tracking data for healthcare decisions, and there are few clinical protocols for making decisions based on patient-reported data. Some doctors worry that storing their patients' self-tracking data puts them at risk of liability if the data could later suggest clues to a missed diagnosis. Healthcare providers may not see more or differently managed data as the primary problem in their clinics, even if the current technology industry rhetoric says that data is the solution to most social problems, including theirs. The process of biomedicalization also means that doctors must compete with app stores and shopping malls for people's attention as they look to lose weight, sleep better, and manage symptoms of chronic diseases, even though widespread belief in the importance of medicine is what created this situation in the first place. Biomedicalization blurs the lines between patient and consumer, and between self-care and doctors' orders.

For some health technology innovators, putting data in the hands of people is itself empowering, can transform the healthcare system, and could make people healthier. For example, healthcare venture capitalist Vinod Khosla says that the purpose of data-driven health innovation should be "to make the consumer the CEO of his own health."[5] Similarly, in the marketing language of the Scanadu Scout, a device that promises to measure vital information by scanning the forehead: "Finally, information about our body is not locked away inside the walls of a hospital," and "Your body's information [is] where it belongs: in your hands."[6] The turn to self-tracking data to solve health problems is not limited to the private sector. The Scottish Government has piloted a mental health self-tracking platform, called Ginsberg, to support people's ability to reflect on their mental health state. It uses a smart diary interface and connection to consumer devices to help people figure out what sorts of circumstances get them down so that they can change those things themselves.

Putting data in the hands of people potentially creates new ways for them to solve their own problems without clinical intervention, and this is a good reason for medical organizations to pursue it. However, data alone cannot create new ways for people to engage in their own health.

While people cannot be expected to participate in medical decision making or change their habits without good information, there seems to be a certain faith that change can come from information alone. The information supplied on the more medical side of the market is perhaps more significant than vague encouragements to engage in "healthy lifestyles," but it is still only information, if it is without support, coaching, or advice. Relying on data alone might not empower in the face of long-standing racial, gender, and class divides that shape healthcare inequalities. Data-wielding patients of the wrong gender or skin color might fare just as badly as before in their attempts to be taken seriously by doctors.

The assumption that the people should have access to the same type of information that doctors have—such as heart rate, blood pressure, blood oxygen saturation— is built into the design of medical self-tracking devices. These home tools can inform people in ways that doctors' visits alone cannot. These things can be measured in a context when something concerning is happening, not days later when an appointment is available. This raises questions about the role of medical expertise. Implicit here is the suggestion that medical interpretation is not always necessary for medical data. Some types of data have long been interpreted by nonprofessionals. People with diabetes learn how make sense of their own glucose levels, for instance. With other types of data, like blood oxygen saturation, there are no widely shared interpretations. With greater power for patients to use data on their own, it has become less clear who will take legal and ethical responsibility for the interpretations and follow-up actions suggested by such data.

Bridging Home and Clinic

Most people spend more time managing their health outside their doctors' offices than inside them. New tools offer the possibility for bridging information that is gathered during doctors' visits with the information from people's daily lives. Tracking at home has long been a part of the toolkit for managing chronic conditions. For tools designed to bridge home and clinic, as opposed to tools designed for the consumer market, information meets medical standards, clinical protocols are considered and designed for, the efficacy is proven, and data protection is in keeping with the standards of health records. Several apps and tools are now being used within clinical settings for tracking mental health or chronic conditions. For example, WellDoc makes a prescription-only, FDA-approved "patient coaching" system for diabetes education and management, helping patients learn how much insulin to take at any particular time.[7] Self-tracking tools and practices can also provide doctors with information about episodes

With greater power for patients to use data on their own, it has become less clear who will take legal and ethical responsibility for the interpretations and follow-up actions suggested by such data.

that may not be apparent through clinical measurement alone. For instance, Ginger.io uses data gathered from smartphones to assess changes in people with serious depression and behavioral problems like schizophrenia. Their website suggests that sensor data can be "a better way to communicate" for your body, a tool that can "help you learn what your body is trying to say," and "a way for you and your care team to hear it." However, the clinical protocols for using this data are only now developing. There is an imperfect relationship between what technologies can do, and how clinicians can handle it.

One way to bridge home and clinic is for doctors to prescribe sensors and trackers, or for medical insurance companies to support their use. One survey found 57 percent of adults said they would be more or much more likely to wear an activity tracker if there were incentives to do so from their insurance companies.[8] A challenge for the designers and makers of these types of self-tracking tools is figuring out how to design for both consumer and medical markets at the same time. There are firms that do this. For example, French device company Withings is working at the boundaries of at-home medicine and consumer electronics. The company has both European and US medical regulators' approval for their products to be sold as home medical devices, such as a connected blood pressure cuff. According to Withings' own research, 42 percent of Withings blood pressure cuff users in the United States who are over sixty years old share their data with their healthcare team.[9] Similarly, Pew Research Center Internet & American Life Project survey results suggested that working with a medical team made self-tracking more likely. That study found that people with chronic conditions were no more likely than average to track diet, weight, or exercise. However, people with more than one chronic condition were *significantly* more likely to track their health indicators or symptoms. This suggests that people who are managing chronic illnesses self-track as part of their ongoing care.[10] Whether or not healthcare teams take this data seriously and incorporate it into their patients' medical records, more companies are seeing opportunities at this boundary.

This raises questions about what needs to be in place before self-tracking and sensor data can be integrated into patient records and used to diagnose and monitor health. Incentives under the U.S. Affordable Care Act support more data-driven medicine, but questions still remain about who will be paid to read and analyze this data, where data will be processed, and what clinical value will come from the data. Data designed to simply inform is likely to fall flat, or be greeted as more work by doctors.

Data can be designed to do other things, however. As Gina's research has shown, self-tracking data can also create opportunities for conversation and connection between patients and their care providers, giving both a chance to educate one another about values and validate personal beliefs, reinforce good practices and behaviors, and fine-tune the goals of treatment plans. The technology itself does not do these things, but opportunities exist, through conversation, to change healthcare decisions ("Should I see a doctor for this?"), build relationships with healthcare providers ("Can we talk about my data?"), and create new opportunities for self-tracking experiments ("Let's see if this is the cause."). One of Gina's collaborators, Dr. Anthony L. Back, an oncologist whose research focuses on patient-doctor communication, says one the new roles for physicians could be to ask their patients what *they* want to do with their own data. As he puts it, if patients are producing, curating, and analyzing their own data, one job for physicians could be to foster "the really complex understanding of how people construct meaning from data. . . . The question for me as a doctor would be how can I contribute to those understandings?"[11] Indeed, new classes of jobs might eventually emerge that are about supporting people as they track health and wellness data, provided resources can be found for such work to be performed. Such work might not be performed by an MD, but could be performed by someone with more expertise in clinical healthcare than a personal data coach or trainer. These opportunities to communicate might, of course, be mitigated by the time constraints of appointments, and they might not play out in the same way when racial, gender or class inequalities are a factor.

Data-Driven Health Innovation and Discovery

So far, we've discussed how self-tracking data could support various types of clinical care. Self-tracking tools can also change how life science research is done at a population level through greater numbers of individual-level experiments and data. One effort emerging is known as digital disease detection, tapping into the data traces from smartphones and computers to improve epidemiology. Self-tracking apps and sensors have the potential for giving new insights to researchers, through passive and continuous data collection, potentially producing better and more information than self-reported surveys or clinical trials. The self-tracking of many people can make ever-larger studies possible. For example, Apple's ResearchKit, a platform for donating data for medical studies, was announced with apps for participating in studies on Parkinson's disease, asthma, diabetes, and heart disease. Within the first twenty-four hours of the announcement of ResearchKit, the heart disease study had 10,000 volunteers, a number that used to take over a year and recruitment through fifty medical centers to reach. The hope is that the large-scale data collection and analysis can lead to new discoveries, and practical ways to tailor approaches to care to individuals.

In QS and many patient advocacy groups, there is a belief that data-driven discoveries in healthcare will not only be done by professional researchers and scientists, but also by ordinary people using their own data from their own experiments. Groups like Cure Together create a "crowdsourced" model of knowledge about diseases, a kind of DIY epidemiology that allows people with chronic conditions to share their own experiences and look for patterns across the group's data. Such approaches show that clinical data may no longer be the purview solely of doctors and clinicians. The question remains whether professional researchers will trust those citizen scientists to interpret their own data or find their claims plausible enough for further testing. Traditionally disempowered communities and communities that have had contentious relationships with medical institutions might struggle to gain that trust.

Nevertheless, there is now support for citizen science from more established institutions like the National Institutes of Health (NIH), which has sponsored workshops on its ethical, legal, and social implications.[12] Jennifer Couch of the National Cancer Institute, speaking for the work of the NIH working group on citizen science, said citizen science methods "have the potential to enable research that really isn't doable in other ways." Her view is that even though they won't ever replace double-blind clinical trials, citizen science experiments and data can still benefit from scientific assessment and rigor. Part of the NIH's interest in supporting citizen science is to make scientific methods and tools more widely available so members of the public can become active participants in science. People are "generally motivated to collect and share health data," said Couch, and the scientific community should figure out ways to use that data and safeguard it legally, ethically, and socially. As she explained, "Anywhere we can see the creativity and capabilities and the unique insights from the public coming to bear in creative ways, we can imagine citizen science approaches being useful for biomedical research."[13]

Integrating insights from self-tracking experiments into the scientific community is one of the ways that self-tracking may change science. To do this, though, these experiments and findings have to cross very different kinds of communities and languages. Working with communities of people who are not scientists means working in the languages of the community, argues Elizabeth Yeampierre, a community organizer for environmental and health justice with Brooklyn's UPROSE organization. Her group works with researchers and scientists to put data collection and analysis tools into the hands of community participants and to build connections between them and experts. Doing so involves teaching scientists to approach communities differently in how they present information as well as teaching scientists to learn and respect that communities come with their own knowledge.[14]

Another example is Cincinnati Children's Chronic Care Network, or C3N, which built a data ecosystem that aims to be meaningful, valuable, and useful for individual (pediatric) patients, their families, and their doctors, as well as for researchers. They use social media to create social support for their pediatric patients with chronic diseases even as they use data from their interactions for research. C3N views data as an opportunity to build communities to help kids with chronic diseases get better. They use a quote from Harvard social media theorist Yochai Benkler on their own website to show their inspiration for this idea: "Once you open the possibility that people are not only using the web as a platform to produce their own individual content, but also to pool their efforts, knowledge, and resources . . . the possibilities for what they can create are astounding."[15] C3N's work shows that n-of-1 data can move in different ways even in a regulated formal healthcare setting *if* it is designed from the ground up to do so. C3N is designing for the different data needs of each of its communities, because, in their words, clinical data is currently "not working for patients who suffer more than they have to. It's not working for their parents who aren't able to participate as part of the care team. It's not working for their doctors who practice based on minimized clinical trials. And, it's not working for researchers who want to make a difference but need access to data."

Eric Topol in *The Creative Destruction of Medicine* uses the phrase "the *n* of 1 to the *n* of billions" to describe this process of scaling up individual-level data. In Topol's view, new types of data will rush in "a new era of medicine, in which each person can be near fully defined at the individual level, instead of how we practice medicine at a population level." By "fully defined" he means that there is an ever-richer picture of each individual person painted by data. Topol is interested in using this rich picture in comparison to what is known at a population level in order to personalize medical treatments. Some bodies might respond differently to different treatments, and he argues if we know more about both the individual ("n of 1") and the aggregate ("n of billions") we can better adapt treatments to particular individuals. The language Topol uses presumes that this richness "fully defines" a person, which is the exact source of consternation for many critics of self-tracking, who believe that people can never be "fully defined" in quantitative data. Medical researchers who are less enthusiastic about these new sources of data point out that the problem of spurious correlation, or an accidental relationship among variables, becomes a bigger problem the more data one has. If you are looking for a needle in a haystack, they argue, why increase the amount of hay?

While data is currently being used in various ways to empower patients, bridge home and clinic, and make new kinds of discoveries, these practices also open up new areas of social uncertainty and debate. Here we identify four, although this is such an emerging, active space that we expect there to be many others to come.

What Makes Data Clinical?

With clinical data, a host of regulations, norms, and professional standards influence what can be considered data and how it can move. Many of the apps developed for commercial digital health have not been tested for their effectiveness and have had little study of how useful they are in clinical settings. Both of these limitations make many doctors skeptical that self-tracking data could ever be clinically useful. One doctor we spoke with, active in QS, put the challenge this way: "Tracking doesn't necessarily actually give you useful information. . . . [Sometimes it's a project] to kind of derive meaning out of things you're tracking that honestly may not have any biologic or medical significance." For doctors "meaning" is rooted in biological or medical significance, even if there are many other kinds of meaning for patients in their own data.[16] Skepticism of n-of-1 data is not universal within the medical community, but doctors and researchers look at the data with particular lenses. They look for whether tests or experiments have what researchers call "face validity," meaning the data makes sense within the context of current biomedical understanding and the measures indicate what people think they indicate. Doctors are used to tailoring dosages and options to individual patients and understand a reasoned trial-and-error approach to individualized treatment plans. But as the QS member and doctor said, practitioners base these on a connection to established medical science. Doctors also care if the data reflects or relates to a set of protocols or actions. They are unlikely to discourage anything that supports healthy behaviors, but are wary of data that does not directly relate to the actions they currently take. For these reasons, there are not currently easy ways of simply folding self-tracking data into more established clinical practices. It is data of a different sort.

More people having more data may very well challenge these orientations, or force doctors to reentrench them in different ways. Advocates like Topol see merit in expanding the definitions of good, medically actionable data beyond the double-blind, randomized, controlled clinical trial, but expansion will not happen without difficult arguments about validity and professional boundary keeping. Advocates for self-tracking data in clinical settings hope that new types of data lead to new ways of doing research and improving personalized medicine. Detractors question whether the data that people collect on their own is valid or any different from other patient-reported outcomes. It could be that such data constitutes another factor in clinical decision making, but not necessarily the most important one and one that is extremely difficult to parse and compare at the population level.

New kinds of clinical data require regulators to consider and clarify distinctions between wellness data and health-care data. The FDA regulates what it calls "mobile medical applications" in cases where smartphones function like a regulated medical device and apps give medical advice. The list of the FDA's examples of mobile medical applications speaks to how extensively mobile devices could eventually power medical tracking: ECG, EKG, stethoscope, audio meter, tremor transducer, and blood oxygen and glucose detection. The agency has said it will "exercise enforcement discretion" for apps and tools for general wellness or for symptom tracking. In other words, the FDA allows most general wellness tools and apps to be largely exempt from an approval process. Much of this regulatory line between regulated health and exempt wellness data depends on the intended uses for the data. An app intended to help patients and their doctors make decisions about treatment would be regulated, while one that encourages "healthy lifestyles" would not. An app intended to measure one's heart rate while hiking likely would not be regulated, but some people may find a way use that data to monitor a medical condition. The FDA uses the hiking heart rate app as an example of one it won't regulate; yet if that same technology were marketed to patients for a medical condition, it becomes a regulated mobile medical app subject to a rigorous approval process.

Some companies have in fact triggered FDA action. Consider the case of uChek by Biosense Technologies, one of the first iPhone apps pulled from the US market in response to action by the FDA. uChek was developed in India as a way to essentially use the capabilities of the iPhone to automate the reading of urine analysis test strips. This device allows for quick, automated field readings of tests that are commonly done in clinics and laboratories. Instead of an expensive piece of equipment, uChek's small and relatively affordable kit makes a person "a walking talking path lab," which is especially important in delivering care to remote parts of rural India. Myshkin Ingawale, Biosense's founder, gave TED talks and was featured in numerous prominent media outlets like *The Guardian* and *Popular Science*.[17] In his TED talk Ingawale demonstrated the app while holding a water bottle full of urine—uChek was not under the radar.

Ingawale says publicly that his mission is to "democratize healthcare," creating alternatives to expensive laboratory equipment, especially important in developing and emerging economy countries. Instead of building a medical device or laboratory equipment from scratch, Ingawale and Biosense leverage commercially available tools, built on the capabilities of smartphones. In his words, "What is the best way to build an advanced electronic device that has high quality imagining, data processing, communication, and interfacing capabilities? Answer: Buy a phone."[18]

Different regulatory regimes among countries have different requirements, which can be a challenge for those seeking to sell technologies in multiple markets. Apple approved uChek for sale in the United States through the iTunes Store. However, in a May 2013 letter, regulators noted that Biosense was marketing something the FDA considered a regulated medical device without having gone through the required approval process. It was the first example of the FDA exercising its regulatory authority over a mobile phone app.[19]

Different companies have different approaches to working in this space and engaging with regulators. Inside Tracker is a dashboard that displays nutritional and lifestyle advice based on the results of clinical bloods tests, and the results disclaim any medical purpose from these medical tests. AlivCore created an ECG heart monitor that attaches to the iPhone. It was first tested on animals and marketed to veterinarians while the company awaited FDA approval and is now marketed directly to consumers. Scanaflo, demoed at the 2015 Consumer Electronics Show, sought FDA approval for a device that will be able to test for several indicators in urine—much like Biosense's uChek. Regulated devices may create shared ground between medical and consumer interpretation of data. However, developing regulatory categories that reflect the emergent types of data and their uses is an ongoing, sometimes contested process.

The clarity of the FDA's mobile medical applications guidance helps companies and nonprofits figure out what they have to do to bring products to market. Sometimes less-established startup companies need further resources to help them navigate the waters or establish clinical efficacy. Biosense, for example, is partnering with pharmaceutical giant Merck on a program in Bangladesh to test uChek for detecting eclampsia among pregnant women. They have also run a crowdfunding campaign to help them pay the fees required for the FDA approval process in the United States.

Some debates are emerging about how to ensure public safety in light of the wide variety of organizations now making medical devices. Startups and patient movements like Nightscout do not have deep pockets to easily absorb costs associated with regulatory processes. Patient communities and user groups might need new ways of working in order to ensure safety, or a regulatory approach that takes into account how they already work, as with open source projects. The documentation of Nightscout's approval process indicates that the FDA is figuring out ways to ensure open source projects can deliver technologies safely, without requiring them to abandon their open source methods for scrutinizing and validating software code. Patient groups like these are better positioned to design for human needs up front, and they may have some valuable input on what constitutes risk and safe practice. Research has shown that in other industries incumbents sometimes influence regulatory processes so that safety is defined in ways designed to keep smaller competitors out. We do not have evidence of that happening in health technology innovation, but it is a well-known phenomenon to be aware of in public debates about what constitutes safe practice. It is also possible that market actors with more resources could more easily provide certain types of safety mechanisms. When the definition of what is considered "clinical" changes, new areas of contestation around safety and medical actionability emerge.

Does Data Change Compliance?

The medical and pharmaceutical research and clinical communities look to self-tracking for new levers for compliance with treatments. "Compliance" is a term of art within medicine, but a problematic one within a long line of sociological and anthropological research. Compliance emphasizes medical expertise over everyday practices in search of what works. It presupposes the solution to a problem is within individual control; it does not consider the social mechanisms or factors that may be root causes of successful or unsuccessful treatment. As a result, people often tune out when credentialed experts pontificate on the righteousness of complying with advice that does not fit their lives.

Doctors may want their patients to follow guidelines for public health reasons—for example, adhering to pharmaceutical treatment plans so as not to lead to drug resistance or to vaccination schedules for the safety of a community. They may want their patients' compliance because the sickest and the poorest of their patients suffer more commonly from diseases preventable by more exercise, better nutrition, and less smoking. These are examples of good reasons why they might want people doing things in prescribed ways.

More fundamental problems of social, political, and economic inequalities might become even more apparent when data is designed to increase compliance. Data alone is likely not enough to force compliance or nudge behavior change. Such self-tracking data might miss social complexity. For example, it might be harder for some people to change behaviors that contribute to preventable diseases. Compliance with drug regimes is harder for people who have less ability to pay for medicines. Some factors—like the predominance of high-calorie, low-nutrient food in certain areas—might be more social than a single behavior change app can fix. Not all requests for compliance are as benign as the reasons already described, and calling a patient "not compliant" can legitimize ignoring patient expertise about why a treatment or a protocol is not workable in their lives and for their social contexts.

Data may or may not change these types of discussions. It could be a new way for clinicians to browbeat patients, but it also could create new ways for clinicians to acknowledge the realities of patients' lives. Dawn Lemanne, for instance, is an oncologist and organizer of the Individual Metabolic Research Group (iMeRG), a group of medical professionals who develop and coordinate single-subject medical studies. She knew that diet and insulin resistance play a crucial role in recovery from breast cancer, so she wondered why one of her breast cancer patients was not regularly testing her glucose. She thought about her patient, "This is your life, why didn't you do it?"[20] She began testing herself, keeping track of how often she succeeded in complying with her own "prescription." In doing so, she discovered just how hard it is to sustain constant testing in the face of life's realities. Her compliance rate was worse than her patient's. As a result Lemanne has more realistic discussions with patients about what compliance entails and better understands why they make the decisions that they do.

Many health technology innovations are built on a concept that people's lives are less complex than what they are. Such companies hold out hope that technology will provide simple solutions for the problems of cost, adherence, and compliance. As one research team put it, "Much of the output of self-monitoring devices and mobile health applications, including the data that they generate, fails to engage people."[21] Is compliance something that can essentially be designed for with an "engaging" design—a game, perhaps, as an incentive you to take your medicines—or is a focus on "engaging design" misplaced when behavior change faces strong social headwinds? Whether a person believes compliance can be solved with design mechanisms for individually used tools depends on how they assume social and individual power works.

Do Medical Apps Address the Wrong People?

In chapter 4, we saw how the consumer market for self-tracking tools generally focuses on relatively younger, healthier, and more technologically sophisticated people compared to the general population. This affects the medical side of the market as well. A Pew study found that while African Americans are actually more likely to self-track, smartphone wellness app users are more likely to be younger, female, and more educated than the general population.[22] As J. C. Herz wrote in *Wired:* "The people who could most benefit from this technology—the old, the chronically ill, the poor—are being ignored."[23] Popular culture critic Anne Helen Peterson called the move of self-tracking from Silicon Valley elites to middle-class, Middle-America moms, neither of whom are the poorest or the sickest.[24]

While there is a tendency for this market to address the already healthy and wealthy, the picture is perhaps more mixed. Biosense started its design for uChek by assuming limited access to medical laboratories and very little wealth. A public conversation should happen about what access to healthcare means and how medical applications on smartphones fit in the social contexts where access to clinical care is a serious problem. These tools can be cheaper than clinical care and ought to be made even cheaper for populations that need them most. However, focusing on technical tools for the poor, in a system also capable of delivering concierge-style medical services for the rich, could be seen as a way to exclude people from access to full healthcare services.

Does Data Lower Costs?

The widely shared faith that data leads to individual change has been taken up in the health insurance industry. Humana, a for-profit health insurance group, is working with a startup called The Activity Exchange, which builds tools based on tracking data to "drive meaningful, intelligent and personalized engagement" of people with their health insurance company.[25] As Bruce Broussard, the CEO of Humana, said, "When people know their numbers they make more effective decisions. . . . Helping them take those steps is the most important thing."[26] Insurance companies like Cigna have started projects that use consumer tracking tools like Fitbit, Bodymedia, and Jawbone Up with the stated goal of encouraging people to be more active. A spokesperson for

Cigna said that this could "bend the cost curve."[27] Sensors also have a role to play in changing the cost equation for geriatric care. One estimate put the cost at retrofitting an elder's home with connected sensors at $2,500, compared to an average annual cost of a nursing facility of more than $81,000.[28] The elderly regularly subvert sensing, however, by intentionally destroying or otherwise hacking sensors to get them to do what they actually need.[29]

We have already seen examples of how the ability to reduce costs might not be as straightforward as the faith in data would suggest, but it might be feasible with care and attention paid to design, behavior change models, and confounding social factors. Data's roles in a complex market in healthcare—a market where actors have conflicting incentives that sometimes do and sometimes do not align with the interests of the public—deserve high levels of scrutiny from the public. If there are indeed cost savings to come through more usage of sensors, the public ought to be asking how much of those costs savings are being returned to them. Again, as with the consumer market, the practices of individual companies differ, but critics like Frank Pasquale argue that transparency makes a difference. How will people know if self-tracking is being used to improve overall population health, or if their data is being used against them? If the cost of opting out is higher insurance premiums, will the ability to opt out only be available in practice to the wealthy?

We have seen examples of how self-tracking data is being integrated into medicine and how this raises new questions and new areas of social contestation. In some corners of medicine, practices are becoming more participatory while in others, hierarchies are asserting themselves anew. Issues of data access, control, privacy, and security are at work in medicine as much as they are in other areas of self-tracking. These common areas of social debate across the various areas of self-tracking we take up in our next, and final, chapter.

FUTURE DIRECTIONS FOR
SELF-TRACKING

We have pointed to some of the social dynamics at work in self-tracking. There we see a picture of elements of surveillance and control mixed with empowerment and playfulness. The future of self-tracking is not fixed. There are key areas of debate about self-tracking that cross the various social worlds, such as technology users and producers, medical communities, patient advocacy groups, and ordinary citizens. In this somewhat speculative conclusion, we offer some final thoughts about the areas of discussion that are emerging among these groups and where these conversations might be headed.

The data collected about our lives touches on our future in the workplace, in the marketplace, and as citizens. Which direction self-tracking ultimately takes depends on the claims that get made about who can access and control data. The future of self-tracking depends on decisions made during design about privacy, data flows, and business models. The future depends on what users of self-tracking technologies decide about what their data means and how they want to use it. Finally, it depends on how regulators handle medical safety and the patchwork of privacy laws that today leaves many people with little recourse to rectify the harms that come to them. The future of self-tracking tools is not just about the next generation of fancy technology for the few. It is fundamentally about what say people have in how knowledge about them is created and disseminated.

The Fight for Data Access

Consider the story of Hugo Campos. Campos became an advocate for patients' rights to access their data when he learned that the manufacturer of his implanted heart defibrillator considered the data the defibrillator generates to be theirs, not his. The company claimed exclusive ownership over the numbers emitting from inside his body, generated by the signals sent from his heart. The company claimed for itself not just the right to monitor his every heartbeat, but the *exclusive* right to control who saw that data and how it was used. It did not deem Campos to be a legitimate user of that data, because he was not a medical professional. Campos, being highly expert on his particular situation, did have some very clear uses for that data. He wanted to learn about the effects of ordinary activities on his heart, such as attending stressful meetings or eating certain foods. Therein lies the hypocrisy of excluding Campos from his own data. Heart patients are widely advised to lead a healthy lifestyle and to "take responsibility" for their health, but when Campos wanted to be able to test the effects of specific lifestyle practices, he was prevented from doing so. Self-tracking technologies are touted by parts of the medical industry as a way for people to "take control" of their health, but when the industry cannot set the terms of what "control" means, people like Campos are greeted with secrecy and paternalism and are actively prevented from watching their own bodies' data in the same way a company can. Indeed, any adjustments to the device or reprogramming to allow him access to his own data would constitute a copyright violation.[1] Campos could not opt out of his heart sending data to the company, unless he made it stop collecting data entirely, which made little sense to him because the data is actually useful.

When his partner changed jobs, Campos was denied access to healthcare. Even though everyday self-care was all that Campos had at the time, the company continued to deny access to this data on the grounds that he was insufficiently expert to care for himself on the basis of it. The raw data, they claimed, was too technical. Indeed, even his doctor (when he had one) could only receive summarized and cleaned versions of the data. Yet eating and exercise are everyday decisions, taken without medical oversight, with effects on the heart, and Campos's medical device produced granular data that could help him think about those decisions.

For Campos, data ownership was not about an obscure legal theory. The data was the stuff of his body, and he wanted it back. As Campos said of all the patients with implanted defibrillators, "Not a single one of these patients is allowed access to their device's data. I am sure you'd agree that this is an objectionable practice and it must be stopped."[2] Campos has been very vocal about his predicament, speaking regularly at patient advocacy events and health technology conferences. Others have rallied around a similar banner of "give me my data!" Campos gained some access to his data after a multiyear public fight. But his individual victory was not a victory for all patients, and it has not yet built the social, legal, and technical mechanisms for making data access more widespread. For others like Campos to get access to their data, there have to be widespread changes to the social and technical infrastructure of medical device data. Accessing data means building the technical pipes, including an appropriate bundle of legal rights for the person who generated that data, and the legal language that governs device usage or alteration and data transmission. Should those most adversely affected by closed data systems have to bear the burden of doing this advocacy work? No individual can do this alone, and many people stand to benefit from systemic change that fuller access would enable.

For Campos, data ownership was not about an obscure legal theory. The data was the stuff of his body, and he wanted it back.

This fight over access to data will continue as long as most companies and doctors default to a position that says data is a proprietary commodity for them to choose whether to make open. Not all institutions see things this way, and ownership rights are not nearly as simple as "you own it or you don't." As with land rights, the right to use, access, share, and sell data can all be separated out and given to different parties. As self-tracking data slowly becomes more integrated into healthcare systems, people will need to speak up in the same way Campos did to ensure their interests are protected. Likewise, there is very little to stop third parties like insurance companies and employers from using self-tracking data to discriminate against the very people who generate it. Clear statements from the public and policy statements about appropriate and inappropriate uses of data could change these practices. We realize that our focus in this book has been on the US healthcare system, and very different dynamics may play out where healthcare is delivered by the public sector and where privacy laws are stronger.

The Fight for Data Privacy and Security

Privacy in self-tracking data is likely to be an ongoing renegotiation in the best of circumstances. Apps, trackers, and wearables will continue to raise privacy and security concerns as technologies evolve and new decisions are made about where data goes.

Some of the challenges for privacy and security for self-tracking tools are technical ones. A 2014 Symantec report on security and privacy of activity trackers found all the devices that they encountered could be easily be turned into surveillance trackers by an unauthorized third party with only inexpensive, off-the-shelf components: "It appears that manufacturers of these devices (including market leaders) have not seriously considered or addressed the privacy implications of wearing their products." They could easily track the locations of people using all of the devices that they discovered in their scans of public areas in two European cities. Most of the transmitting apps that they discovered in their scans even lacked a privacy policy. The apps that they found sent user data to an average of five different Internet domains, meaning that up to five different companies got the data straight from the users' smartphones. Few customers were aware of this.[3]

Regulators are beginning to weigh in on this issue. The chair of the US Federal Trade Commission (FTC), Edith Ramirez, has called for more attention to be paid to the data protection of self-tracking devices. In her speech at the Consumer Electronics Show (CES) in 2015, she said: "In the not-too-distant future, many, if not most, aspects of our everyday lives will be digitally observed and stored. That data trove will contain a wealth of revealing information that, when patched together, will present a deeply personal and startlingly complete picture of each of us—one that includes details about our financial circumstances, our health, our religious preferences, and our family and friends." Ramirez continued with a glimpse into the dystopian ways that data could be used against consumers, without transparency in how the data is shared:

> Your smart TV and tablet may track whether you watch the history channel or reality television, but will your TV-viewing habits be shared with prospective employers or universities? Will they be shared with data brokers, who will put those nuggets together with information collected by your parking lot security gate, your heart monitor, and your smart phone? And will this information be used to paint a picture of you that you will not see but that others will—people who might make decisions about whether you are shown ads for organic food or junk food, where your call to customer service is routed, and what offers of credit and other products you receive?

The following year at CES, Ramirez went even further, saying that she didn't trust her own data to the companies who make activity trackers and instead relied on an old-fashioned pedometer that isn't connected to the Internet.[4] That such a future could be reasonably predicted at an industry conference by a regulator should concern consumers. The fact that much of this future is already with us should concern us all. Will the data, Ramirez asks, be used to provide services to customers or will it be used in ways that are inconsistent with "consumers' expectations and relationship with a company?" Here we see a signal from the US federal government that contextual integrity and the expectations about social relationships between people and the companies they buy from do matter. These questions are particularly important for health and wellness data, but they also raise more general questions about people's rights to the data that they generate in a data-driven culture.

Not only could your data be used against you if handled improperly, it could also be used to find you. Research by computer scientists continues to show that even anonymized data can be identified and attributed to specific individuals. A pioneering researcher in this field, Harvard Professor Latanya Sweeney, was part of a team that was able to link names and contact information to the publically available profiles in the Personal Genome Project, a project where people share their data from genome sequencing. The "reidentification" of anonymous data exploited known weaknesses in large-scale demographic data sets. By mining public records for the seemingly innocuous information of birth date, gender, and zip code, Sweeney's team correctly identified 84–97 percent of the time anonymous profiles that contained demographic along with genetic and medical information. If data from just a few pieces of demographic information (which is less strongly protected under US law than personally identifiable information and health records) can identify someone, imagine what adding genetic information or disease conditions could mean for privacy risks in large-scale shared and pooled data.[5]

Both technical and legal solutions have a role to play here. As frightening as large data sets can be, we do not live in a world where they are avoidable. Many important social functions depend on large data sets, such as medical research and public social science surveys. There is a concern here that researchers or companies might stockpile data because others are doing it, not because of a genuine need for particular data. Legal, rather than technical, solutions might have a stronger effect on that practice.

Security technologies also need to evolve to facilitate data exchange where appropriate, and companies need to take the time to build them into their systems to ensure that data sets of this magnitude do not get broken into. The traditional "lock it down" approach to security does not work in a data-rich world where moving data around can have positive benefits. Security technologies can also help ensure that when data is shipped out, it is shipped to the right person and not intercepted in between. Technical approaches can reduce the risk of unintended effects of appropriate data exchanges, but they are not enough.

Clearly technology cannot fix the inherent way that data leaves traces of people, and that is where the law can step in. Policymakers are beginning to question whether our frameworks for consent and notification can still work in a data-saturated world, although privacy activists disagree that these frameworks are irreparably broken.[6] Just because companies and researchers can technically de-anonymize anonymous data does not mean that they should or be legally allowed to do so. There could be (as there is in the United Kingdom) legal sanctions against reidentifying individuals in anonymized data sets. This acknowledges that data "exhaust" puts everyone at risk to some extent, but criminalizes actions that could bring people harm. Where technology cannot prevent people from acting poorly, policy can do so.

Another potential tool in the fight for privacy is transparency. Even if transparency does not come via legislative means, researchers, journalists, and like-minded industry actors can encourage greater transparency in how data is controlled by creating detailed accounts of where exactly data goes, and under what legal and technical conditions. In the same spirit, the radio program "Planet Money" purchased a "toxic asset" and followed it through its subsequent sale and resale to help the public understand how toxic assets crashed economies. Similar data-tracing exercises can be difficult, but some projects have already begun to appear that make apparent who is buying records of your Internet data trail. Audit studies of algorithms show how companies manipulate social media data, and within Quantified Self some community members have attempted to document data flows.[7] Technical systems that ensure that data provenance is preserved could help support such transparency.

The Legal and Regulatory Questions about Data

The law around self-tracking data is also developing. How data can be used in court, by employers, by marketers, or by insurance companies has yet to be figured out. This issue carries enormous civil liberties implications. Civil liberties groups and racial justice organizations are fighting for what one document calls the "Civil Rights Principles for the Era of Big Data." At issue is "high-tech profiling," in which "new surveillance tools and data gathering techniques that can assemble detailed information about any person or group create a heightened risk of profiling and discrimination."[8] Groups like the New America Foundation's Open Technology Institute, the American Civil Liberties Union, and the NAACP are signatories. The data-driven analytics culture has a significant capacity to lead to "digital redlining," using data for "new forms of discrimination and predatory practices" in health, as well as housing, employment, credit, and the consumer marketplace, a White House report on big data and privacy found.[9]

It is increasingly difficult to ensure the personal privacy of linked health data but important to do so in light of the potential gains to research and treatment. Self-tracking data may soon be linked to other data to suggest the onset of symptoms or conditions earlier than reported symptoms. A change in the number of daily steps, a detection of small movements that could indicate tremors, and even differences in Internet search patterns can all theoretically be used to help make diagnoses and some companies are already working on this. However, it will be an enormous challenge to protect this type of data, especially as it becomes possible to infer more personal information from seemingly innocuous data. As a White House report put it, "Traditionally, health data privacy policies have sought to protect the identity of individuals whose information is being shared and analyzed. But increasingly, data about groups or categories of people will be used to identify diseases prior to or very early after the onset of clinical symptoms."[10] Data collected in doctors' offices are afforded one type of protection, but we do not have in place the legal frameworks that offer protections to similar data gathered from our smartphones, web searches, and digital devices.

Our health data privacy policies have been based upon protecting identifiable information about individuals. But what about data for groups or families? Our choice about sharing our genetic information does not solely expose us, it also potentially identifies and implicates our biological

Data collected in doctors' offices are afforded one type of protection, but we do not have in place the legal frameworks that offer protections to similar data gathered from our smartphones, web searches, and digital devices.

parents and children. While some protections are in place in the United States through the Genetic Information Nondiscrimination Act (or GINA), those protections extend just to health insurance and employment discrimination, and not to the whole host of other types of potential harms that come from the inappropriate uses of this data. Microbiome data is another type of data that shows similarities among people who live together or were raised together. Microbiome data may reveal as much about one's family and neighborhood as it does about oneself.

Nor do we yet have legal protection for data that identifies us, not in name, but "in all likelihood." Kate Crawford and Jason Schultz call this a potential for "predictive privacy harms." They have noted that while there are laws in the United States that cover the loss of personally identifiable information, there is no case law to cover the situation that with enough data your identity could be inferred with high likelihood from a combination of variables (say, the combination of zip code, birth month, gender, and make of car leading to one particular person).[11] This is far from a theoretical risk. Several states already routinely sell their records on hospitalizations to private companies, and researchers connected these records to specific individuals in up to 43 percent of cases merely through using publicly available data.[12] The risk of predictive privacy harms is increased by the more extensive collection of data across many spheres of life. But hospitals' long-standing practice of selling data also increases that risk. The lack of clear policies and regulations for data privacy in the United States makes it difficult to hold companies legally liable for stronger data protection.

How self-tracking data will "count" in a court of law is still being decided. Police in Lancaster, Pennsylvania, used Fitbit data to discredit a woman's story of an attack and to charge her with making a false police report.[13] The company Vivametrica markets its services preparing activity tracker data for use in personal injury cases, or what one critic called "quantified self incrimination."[14] Vivametrica says, "Wearable technology is a tool that attorneys ought to embrace because facts don't lie. By leveraging wearables data, lawyers can bring more accuracy to cases, resulting in greater credibility."[15] One attorney called wearable devices a "black box" for the human body, creating ways to measure injury claims, for example, and the data is beginning to be used that way.[16] Of course, throughout this book we have seen plenty of cases where data is far short of "facts" that "don't lie." Sensors yield spurious spikes, data goes missing, and the contextual information needed to make sense of the data can't come from the device itself. Self-tracking tools work as consumer devices when people have control over them and over how their data is used. If such data becomes common as a form of legal evidence, there will be a chill in the market for these tools.

Future Directions for Technology Innovation

Smaller startups have made great gains in consumer wellness and can bring design and technology expertise to regulated medical markets through new kinds of tools. However, a mix of regulatory processes and agencies means that relatively few startup companies have embraced the challenges of designing for more highly regulated arenas like hospitals and home healthcare.

The technical standards that allow people and companies to collaborate across multiple devices, platforms, and data types are still in development. Some companies' businesses rely on the ability to prevent customers from taking their data and leaving, while other companies would benefit from a more open ecosystem that allows users to choose among the services and companies that can use their data. Currently, companies that provide behavior-change coaching use data from other devices. Open APIs enable firms to build on each other's systems. There is now emerging a small cadre of startups positioning themselves to mediate data among companies and users, so it appears that a degree of openness and interoperability is taking shape, even if the distinction between clinical and nonclinical data creates challenges in the process. As we have seen, getting data out of medical device ecosystems and combining it with other self-tracking data can make an enormous difference for the patients who are managing chronic conditions.

While discussions about technical standards for data interoperability bore some people to tears, interoperability matters because it facilitates people's ability to generate innovations, examples of which we have seen in this book.

Debates about Health and Equity

If self-tracking is to help the sickest and the poorest, then tools will need to be designed for those communities in mind. Analysts are already calling the activity tracker market crowded, even though to us this oversight is fairly glaring. In this book we have seen how tools often do not draw on the science of behavior change in its fullest capacity, or take into account the very real social problems that create health issues in the first place. They too often rely instead on a simple notion that works for highly motivated people, "data leads to knowledge and knowledge leads to change."

There are very real questions about who, realistically, is best positioned to fill this gap. Markets are great at solving certain kinds of problems, and rapid innovation is happening in profit-driven, consumer-facing health and wellness data. In other areas of life, attempts to resolve social problems through consumer markets have been met with mixed results. For example, many critics have complained that designing consumer goods for the "bottom of the pyramid"—i.e., the poor in developing countries—has proved even more exploitative than no intervention at all, while creating a veneer of charitability for the firms involved. Markets are an undeniable part of civic life, and firms will continue to have a role to play. However, we should all think about which actors can best align their interests with civic interests, delivering goods and services that meet people's needs beyond where needs simply intersect with profitability. Grassroots projects like Nightscout are clear examples of citizens intervening when the market is not meeting their needs. Whether that unpaid work should be shouldered by families or whether there is enough public interest to merit policies that support that activity is a debate worth having.

The design choices that companies make about what data is worth collecting will shape what data is available for clinical practice and medical research. Organizations like Validic and Open mHealth work to find ways to assign clinical definitions to new data types as they emerge from new sensors and applications. If there is to be a greater role for self-tracking data able to motivate actions, care teams, protocols, and treatments in the social world of regulated healthcare, then more work has to happen to translate self-tracking data into clinical realms. This might require companies to ensure that there is room for others to use data in new ways or to get more involved in conversations about data commensurability.

Whether there ultimately will be more public involvement in biomedical research as a result of self-tracking data depends on what the public thinks about the goals of medical research and their confidence in the contextual integrity and privacy of their data. Some self-trackers hold dear the idea that data is uniquely individual, and might not want their data to be forced into commensurability with others. Researchers who move between n-of-1 sensing and population-level knowledge must wrestle with the heterogeneity of self-tracking data. Some life sciences and medical researchers will follow the call of Eric Topol and others to try to draw a totalizing, individualized picture of health from both self-tracking and other kinds of medical data. Others will design tools and protocols for combining individual-level data with greater social and contextual knowledge. The feasibility and desirability of this is likely to continue to be an area of social contestation.

The Fights over Meaning

Datafication means that societies privilege data, and data-driven outcomes, over other kinds of knowing. When data mediates so many things, control over the meanings of data is a type of power. In this book we have seen cases where people assert for themselves high levels of control over what their data means, often by going off-script when the apps do not suit their context. When app companies get their users' social context wrong, as they often do in trying to design for the widest possible market or to square commercial imperatives with customers' needs, they can create problems more serious than an underwhelming product. Tone deaf or ill-conceived meanings for data can cause real harm.

One app user, Kim McAuliffe, has written movingly about these harms. McAuliffe, a game designer in Seattle, had been using fertility tracking apps in the course of trying to get pregnant. She tested positive for pregnancy, but subsequently lost the baby. This was a deeply painful loss for her. While pregnant, she had downloaded multiple pregnancy tracking apps, all of which made design choices that made her question whether any actual women had been in the design process: "All of them had a disturbing similarity with the assumption that pregnant women can only properly grasp the size of a growing fetus as compared to food items." This assumption perhaps could be labeled unfortunate, and caused no real harm to her. However, she received weeks of "unwanted mail about formula for a baby you'll never have, which is a stab in the heart every time 'unsubscribe' fails to work." As if being made to revisit trauma through opt-out marketing were not bad enough, she returned to her fertility tracking app only to find that they had deleted all of her data—over a full year's worth—once she changed her status to "pregnant." The app did this so that the previous data did not influence their algorithm's predictions about fertility after a nine-month pregnancy, which they assumed would be the case for most people. The company, she reports, has since changed this practice and eventually found the data for her.[17] Her experience of having to fight to get data back—data that reflects a painful experience, but also would be helpful in the future—reflects just how vulnerable we are to app makers' decisions about what data indicates about a person.

Every time we glance at our smartphones to see how many steps we've taken is an opportunity to ask questions about how we want to make sense of our worlds, our experiences, and our bodies, and what we want to say to the companies that make it their business to help us do those things. The line between ourselves and our data is where we choose to draw it. We can insist on a clear and meaningful distinction between things that are counted for good reasons, and things that should never be measured and quantified at all. In this, there can be room for the failed experiment. People in QS have grappled with experiments about areas of life that are not easily quantifiable, or are problematic to quantify, and about medical conditions for which neither science nor self-tracking offer clear treatments.

Gracious ways of approaching feelings, emotions, and the ineffable, while recognizing biophysical traces in play, are rarely on offer in the self-tracking market. It could

The line between ourselves and our data is where we choose to draw it.

be that the market is in a poor position to deliver them, but that does not make them inconceivable. Linda Stone, who coined the phrase "continuous partial attention" to describe hyper-media-saturated and fractured lives, describes how she looked to control debilitating long-term pain from trigeminal neuralgia: "My mind and body needed to be friends. They needed to be partners in health. There might be a way to contribute to that through technology, but quantified self technologies did not feel kind, and I wanted to do things for my body that were kind." She found that when the data is troubling and chronic pain is an issue, streams of health data can be frustrating and overwhelming, and she looked to techniques instead that helped her with what she calls "the essential self," including meditation, biofeedback, and an increasing a feeling of embodiment.[18] The experiences of many in QS and elsewhere suggest that there is still a future for using technology to bring us back into awareness of our senses, and to do so in the kindest possible ways, but it is a future that needs to be fought for.

Future Directions for You

Hugo Campos began his fight not just because he was wronged, but also because he knew what he could do with his data if he were given it. We hope that readers have a sense of this too, from some of the stories we share in this book. There is much to learn from the people who have advocated for self-tracking, even though the social systems that surround self-tracking data have numerous problems. Our personal experiences in self-tracking, in awareness of these broader social dynamics, have led us to believe that data can alternate between scary *and* empowering, overwhelming *and* manageable, informative *and* confusing. Learning how to keep track can provide grounded reasons for when *not* to track and a basis for asking much tougher questions of those who would coerce or force us to track.

There is room for both play and resistance in data, as data artists and self-tracking enthusiasts show. Activist communities focused on patients' rights to their data inspire us to hope for more. Both kinds of communities are excellent examples of ways that people have comprehended the logics and cultures of big data for what they are while seeking to change them. Their practices show that data's uncertainties and proliferations are not deterministic, and in some cases can be turned into assets, controlled by ordinary people themselves. Companies and the medical profession design their values into devices they deliver, but that does not give them right to the last word, the last experiment, or the last data set.[19]

There are still many choices that communities and societies must make about what self-tracking practices mean. We hope our readers will see from this book that self-tracking tools can be made and remade with your involvement. We hope that these stories of how people worked with their own data have given you ways to consider how data does or does not play a role in your own lives. We think a future of self-tracking that supports people asking and answering their *own* questions with their *own* data is a future worth fighting for.

1 An Introduction to Self-Tracking

1. IDC, "IDC Forecasts Worldwide Shipments of Wearables to Surpass 200 Million in 2019," http://www.idc.com/getdoc.jsp?containerId=prUS41100116, accessed March 29, 2016.

2. Nora Young, *The Virtual Self* (Toronto: McClelland & Stewart, 2012).

3. For further discussion of healthism, see Julie Guthman, *Weighing In: Obesity, Food Justice, and the Limits of Capitalism* (Berkeley: University of California Press, 2011).

4. Benjamin Franklin's self-examination quote is from his autobiography. See "The Electric Ben Franklin," http://www.ushistory.org/franklin/autobiography/page41.htm, accessed August 22, 2015.

5. Lee Humphreys, Phillipa Gill, Balachander Krishnamurthy, and Elizabeth Newbury, "Historicizing New Media: A Content Analysis of Twitter," *Journal of Communication* 63 (2013): 413–431.

6. Adele E. Clarke, "Biomedicalization," in *The Wiley Blackwell Encyclopedia of Health, Illness, Behavior, and Society* (Hoboken, NJ: John Wiley & Sons 2003): 137–142.

7. Mika Pantzar and Minna Ruckenstein, "The Heart of Everyday Analytics: Emotional, Material and Practical Extensions in Self-Tracking Market," *Consumption Markets & Culture* 18 (2015): 92–109. See also Minna Ruckenstein, "Visualized and Interacted Life: Personal Analytics and Engagements with Data Doubles," *Societies* 4 (2014): 68–84.

8. The study of lead users is Eun Kyoung Choe, Nicole B. Lee, Bongshin Lee, Wanda Pratt, and Julie A. Kientz, "Understanding Quantified-Selfers' Practices in Collecting and Exploring Personal Data," 32nd Annual ACM Conference on Human Factors in Computing Systems (New York: ACM, 2014), 1143–1152. The national study is Susannah Fox and Maeve Duggan, "Tracking for Health" (Washington, DC: Pew Research Center Internet & American Life Project, 2013).

9. Sara Watson, "Living with Data: Personal Data Uses of the Quantified Self" (MSc thesis, University of Oxford, 2013), http://www.scribd.com/doc/172418320/Living-With-Data-Personal-Data-Uses-of-the-Quantified-Self, accessed December 15, 2015.

10. Ian Li, Anind Dey, and Jodi Forlizzi, "A Stage-Based Model of Personal Informatics Systems," in *Proceedings of the SIGCHI Conference on Human Factors in Computing Systems* (New York: ACM, 2010), 557–566.

11. PricewaterhouseCoopers, "The Wearable Future," 2014, http://www.pwc.com/us/en/technology/publications/wearable-technology.html, accessed December 14, 2015.

12. Economist Intelligence Unit, PricewaterhouseCoopers, "Emerging mHealth: Paths for Growth," June 7, 2012, https://www.pwc.com/gx/en/healthcare/mhealth/assets/pwc-emerging-mhealth-chart-pack.pdf, accessed December 14, 2015.

13. Jody Rank, "Platform Wars for the Quantified Self," October 20, 2014, http://research.gigaom.com/report/platform-wars-for-the-quantified-self, accessed November 15, 2014.

14. PricewaterhouseCoopers, "The Wearable Future," 17.

15. One example is Deborah Lupton, "The Digitally Engaged Patient: Self-Monitoring and Self-Care in the Digital Health Era," *Social Theory & Health* 11 (2013): 256–270. Another is Melissa Gregg, *Work's Intimacy* (Hoboken, NJ: John Wiley & Sons, 2013).

16. One example is Askild Matre Aasarød, "A Dislocated Gut Feeling: An Analysis of Cyborg Relations in Diabetes Self-Care" (MA thesis, Aarhus University, 2012). Another is Natasha Dow Schüll, *Keeping Track: Personal Informatics, Self-Regulation, and the Data-Driven Life* (New York: Farrar, Straus, and Giroux, forthcoming).

17. Linda Stone, "A Discussion of Essential Self Technologies," April 30, 2014, http://lindastone.net/2014/04/30/a-discussion-of-essential-self-technologies/, accessed December 14, 2015.

18. Adrian Mackenzie, *Transductions: Bodies and Machines at Speed* (London: A&C Black, 2006).

19. Deborah Lupton, "Self-Tracking Modes: Reflexive Self-Monitoring and Data Practices," last modified August 19, 2014, http://dx.doi.org/10.2139/ssrn.2483549, accessed December 14, 2015.

20. Carl Cederström and André Spicer, *The Wellness Syndrome* (London: Polity, 2015).

21. For a fuller description of communities of practice, see Penelope Eckert, "Communities of Practice," *Encyclopedia of Language and Linguistics* 2 (2006): 683–685.

22. Charles Kadushin, *The American Intellectual Elite* (Boston: Little, Brown, 1974).

23. Tim Ferriss, "The First-Ever Quantified Self Notes," http://fourhourworkweek.com/2013/04/03/the-first-ever-quantified-self-notes-plus-lsd

-as-cognitive-enhancer/, accessed March 7, 2015. See also the post by Gary Wolf after that first meeting, "Why? | Quantified Self," http://quantifiedself .com/2008/09/but-why/, accessed March 7, 2015.

24. Kristen Barta and Gina Neff, "Technologies for Sharing: Lessons from Quantified Self about the Political Economy of Platforms," *Information, Communication & Society* 19 (2016): doi: 10.1080/1369118X.2015.1118520.

25. Gary Wolf, "The Data-Driven Life." *New York Times*, April 28, 2010, http://www .nytimes.com/2010/05/02/magazine/02self-measurement-t.html, accessed December 14, 2015.

2 What Is at Stake?

1. Minna Ruckenstein, "Visualized and Interacted Life: Personal Analytics and Engagements with Data Doubles," *Societies* 4 (2014): 68–84.

2. Nanna Gorm and Irina Shklovski, "Steps, Choices, and Moral Accounting: Observations from a Step-Counting Campaign in the Workplace," CSCW '16, San Francisco, 2016.

3. Evgeny Morozov, *To Save Everything, Click Here: The Folly of Technological Solutionism* (New York: PublicAffairs, 2013).

4. Jacqueline Wheelwright, "Self-Tracking for Autoimmune Mastery," November 8, 2015, https://vimeo.com/144678614, accessed November 22, 2015.

5. Seth Roberts, "Reaction Time as a Measure of Health," January 9, 2014, http://blog.sethroberts.net/2014/01/09/reaction-time-as-a-measure-of -health/, accessed November 22, 2015.

6. Seth Roberts, "Lessons of This Blog (2nd of 2)," December 27, 2013, http:// blog.sethroberts.net/2013/12/27/lessons-of-this-blog-2nd-of-2/, accessed December 16, 2015.

7. Daniel Rosenberg, "Data before the Fact," in *Raw Data Is an Oxymoron*, ed. Lisa L. Gitelman (Cambridge, MA: MIT Press, 2013), 15–40.

8. Ernesto Ramirez, "Talking Data with Your Doc: The Patient," March 29, 2012, http://quantifiedself.com/2012/03/talking-data-with-your-doc/, accessed August 9, 2015.

9. "Quantified Self Public Health Symposium," April 3, 2014, http://quantified self.com/symposium/Symposium-2014/, accessed November 22, 2015.

10. Lorraine Daston and Peter Galison, *Objectivity* (New York: Zone Books, 2007).

11. Ernesto Ramirez, "QS Access: Ian Eslick on Personal Experimentation," January 21, 2015, http://quantifiedself.com/2015/01/qs-access-ian-eslick-personal -experimentation/, accessed November 22, 2015.

12. Brittany Fiore-Gartland and Gina Neff, "Communication, Mediation, and the Expectations of Data: Data Valences across Health and Wellness Communities," *International Journal of Communication* 9 (2015): 1466–1484, http://ijoc.org/index.php/ijoc/article/view/2830, accessed November 22, 2015.

13. David F. Carr, "Quantified Self Should Be about Health, Not Ego," *InformationWeek*, September 25, 2014, http://www.informationweek.com/healthcare/patient-tools/quantified-self-should-be-about-health-not-ego-/a/d-id/1316069, accessed November 22, 2015.

14. Annemarie Mol, *The Logic of Care: Health and the Problem of Patient Choice* (London: Routledge, 2008).

15. Brittany Fiore-Gartland and Gina Neff, "Disruption and the Political Economy of Self-Tracking Data," in *Quantified: Biosensors in Everyday Life*, ed. Dawn Nafus (Cambridge, MA: MIT Press, 2016), 101–122.

16. Ernesto Ramirez, "The DIY Pancreas: An Access Conversation with Dana Lewis & Scott Leibrand," February 17, 2015, https://medium.com/access-matters/do-it-yourself-diabetes-bd1ea1adf034, accessed November 22, 2015.

17. Brad Millington, "Smartphone Apps and the Mobile Privatization of Health and Fitness," *Critical Studies in Media Communication* 31 (2014): 479–493, doi:10.1080/15295036.2014.973429.

18. Helen Nissenbaum, *Privacy in Context: Technology, Policy, and the Integrity of Social Life* (Redwood City, CA: Stanford University Press, 2009).

19. Bill Maurer, "Principles of Descent and Alliance for Big Data," in *Data, Now Bigger and Better!*, ed. Tom Boellstorff and Bill Maurer (Chicago: Prickly Paradigm Press, 2015), 67–86.

3   Making Sense of Data

1. Natasha Dow Schüll, "The Folly of Technological Solutionism: An Interview with Evgeny Morozov," September 9, 2013, http://www.publicbooks.org/interviews/the-folly-of-technological-solutionism-an-interview-with-evgeny-morozov , accessed December 14, 2015.

2. "Amelia Greenhall on Gold Star Experiments," December 31, 2012, http://quantifiedself.com/2012/12/amelia-greenhall-on-gold-star-experiments/, accessed December 14, 2015.

3. Susan Greenhalgh, "Weighty Subjects: The Biopolitics of the US War on Fat," *American Ethnologist* 39 (2012): 471–487.

4. Whitney Erin Boesel, "The Woman vs. the Stick," September 20, 2012, http://thesocietypages.org/cyborgology/2012/09/20/the-woman-vs-the-stick-mindfulness-at-quantified-self-2012/, accessed December 14, 2015.

5. Robin Barooah, "I Am Broken, or I Can Learn," September 18, 2011, http://quantifiedself.com/2011/09/robin-barooah-i-am-broken-or-i-can-learn/, accessed November 15, 2015.

6. Attributed to QS community member Seth Roberts. See Andrew Gelman, "Seth Roberts," April 30, 2014, http://andrewgelman.com/2014/04/30/seth-roberts/, accessed December 14, 2015.

7. Kevin Kelly, "Closing Keynote," Quantified Self 2012 Global Conference, Palo Alto, CA, https://vimeo.com/56082231, accessed March 9, 2015.

8. "Feelspace," http://www.feelspace.de/, accessed December 14, 2015.

9. "Stephen Cartwright," http://www.stephencartwright.com, accessed December 14, 2015.

10. Rob Walker, "How to Pay Attention: 20 Ways to Win the War against Seeing," December 18, 2014, https://medium.com/re-form/how-to-pay-attention-4751adb53cb6, accessed December 14, 2015.

11. Daniela Rosner, "Say I Love You with Mapping," February 9, 2015, https://medium.com/re-form/say-i-love-you-with-mapping-a386df308d78, accessed December 14, 2015.

12. Dawn Nafus and Jamie Sherman, "This One Does Not Go Up to 11: The Quantified Self Movement as an Alternative Big Data Practice," *International Journal of Communication* 8 (2014): 1784–1794.

13. Nick Feltron created beautiful annual reports on minute details about his everyday life. See http://feltron.com/, accessed December 14, 2015.

14. Walker, "How to Pay Attention."

15. Anne Wright, "Breaking Free from the Tyranny of the Norm," July 22, 2014, http://quantifiedself.com/2014/07/anne-wright-breaking-free-tyranny-norm/, accessed December 14, 2015.

16. Anne Wright, *The BodyTrack Project* (Berlin: Springer, forthcoming).

17. Joseph Dumit, "Illnesses You Have to Fight to Get: Facts as Forces in Uncertain, Emergent Illnesses," *Social Science & Medicine* 62 (2006): 577–590.

18. Alexandra Carmichael, "Mark Drangsholt on Tracking a Heart Rhythm Disorder," April 2, 2012, http://quantifiedself.com/2012/04/mark-drangsholt/, accessed December 14, 2015.

19. B. J. Fogg, "Forget Big Change, Start with a Tiny Habit," http://tedxtalks.ted.com/video/Forget-big-change-start-with-a/, accessed December 14, 2015.

20. Charles Duhigg, *The Power of Habit: Why We Do What We Do in Life and Business* (New York: Random House, 2012).

21. Jeremy Dean, *Making Habits, Breaking Habits: Why We Do Things, Why We Don't, and How to Make Any Change Stick* (Boston: Da Capo Lifelong, 2013).

22. Whitney Erin Boesel, "By Whom, For Whom? Science, Startups, and the Quantified Self," October 17, 2013, http://thesocietypages.org/cyborgology/2013/10/17/by-whom-for-whom-science-startups-and-quantified-self/, accessed December 14, 2015.

23. Sophie Day, Celia Lury, and Nina Wakeford, "Number Ecologies: Numbers and Numbering Practices," *Distinktion: Scandinavian Journal of Social Theory* 15 (2014): 123–154.

24. Gerd Gigerenzer and Adrian Edwards, "Simple Tools for Understanding Risks: From Innumeracy to Insight," *British Medical Journal* 327 (2003): 741–744.

25. Data Sense is a research prototype (not a commercial product) built by a research team at Intel co-led by Dawn.

26. Improvements in machine vision software will make this task easier over time, provided technology developers make these tools available for self-tracking applications.

27. Ana Viseu and Lucy Suchman, "Wearable Augmentations: Imaginaries of the Informed Body," in *Technologized Images, Technologized Bodies*, ed. Jeanette Edwards, Penny Harvey, and Peter Wade (New York and Oxford: Berghahn Books, 2010), 161–184.

4   Self-Tracking and the Technology Industry

1. Evgeny Morozov, *To Save Everything, Click Here: The Folly of Technological Solutionism* (New York: PublicAffairs, 2013), xi.

2. Berg Insight, n.d., "Connected Wearables," http://www.berginsight.com/ReportPDF/ProductSheet/bi-cw1-ps.pdf, accessed November 22, 2015.

3. Sam Colt, "Investors Are Massively Underestimating the Apple Watch," November 19, 2014, http://uk.businessinsider.com/investors-are-massively-underestimating-the-apple-watch-2014-11, accessed December 27, 2014.

4. Malay Gandhi and Teresa Wang, "Rock Health Digital Health Funding Year in Review 2014," January 1, 2015, http://www.slideshare.net/RockHealth/rock-health-2014-year-in-review-funding-1, accessed November 22, 2015.

5. Dawn Nafus and Jamie Sherman, "This One Does Not Go Up to 11: The Quantified Self Movement as an Alternative Big Data Practice," *International Journal of Communication* 8 (2014): 1784–1794, http://ijoc.org/index.php/ijoc/article/view/2170, accessed November 22, 2015.

6. Yuliya Grinberg, "Destination: You," October 6, 2015, http://blog.castac.org/2015/10/06/destination-you/, accessed December 14, 2015.

7. Ian Hacking, *The Taming of Chance* (Cambridge, UK: Cambridge University Press, 1990).

8. Morozov, *To Save Everything*.

9. Harry McCracken and Lev Grossman, "Google vs. Death," *Time*, September 30, 2014, http://time.com/574/google-vs-death/, accessed November 22, 2015.

10. Dawn Nafus, "Design for X: Prediction and the Embeddedness (or not) of Research in Technology Production," in *Subversion, Conversion, Development: Cross-Cultural Knowledge Exchange and the Politics of Design*, ed. James Leach and Lee Wilson (Cambridge, MA: MIT Press, 2013), 201–222.

11. Parmy Olson and Aaron Tilley, "The Quantified Other: Nest and Fitbit Chase a Lucrative Side Business," April 17, 2014, http://www.forbes.com/sites/parmyolson/2014/04/17/the-quantified-other-nest-and-fitbit-chase-a-lucrative-side-business/, accessed November 22, 2015.

12. Matthew Herper, "Surprise! With $60 Million Genentech Deal, 23andMe Has a Business Plan," January 6, 2015, http://www.forbes.com/sites/matthewherper/2015/01/06/surprise-with-60-million-genentech-deal-23andme-has-a-business-plan/, accessed December 13, 2015.

13. Frank Pasquale, *The Black Box Society* (Cambridge, MA: Harvard University Press, 2015).

14. The White House, "Big Data: Seizing Opportunities, Preserving Values: Interim Progress Report," February 2015, https://www.whitehouse.gov/sites/default/files/docs/20150204_Big_Data_Seizing_Opportunities_Preserving_Values_Memo.pdf, accessed December 13, 2015.

15. Hanna Wallach, "Big Data, Machine Learning, and the Social Sciences," December 19, 2014, https://medium.com/@hannawallach/big-data-machine-learning-and-the-social-sciences-927a8e20460d#.5a2igmr4g, accessed December 13, 2015.

16. Gandhi and Wang, "Rock Health Digital Health Funding Year in Review 2014," 14.

17. Jonah Comstock, "NBA Players Start Wearing Wearable Health Trackers," February 19, 2014, http://mobihealthnews.com/30109/nba-players-start-wearing-wearable-health-trackers/, accessed November 22, 2015.

18. Olivia Solon, "Wearable Technology Creeps into the Workplace," *Bloomberg Business*, August 6, 2015, http://www.bloomberg.com/news/articles/2015-08-07/wearable-technology-creeps-into-the-workplace, accessed December 14, 2015.

19. See Eric Wicklund, "Smartwatches Are Missing a Crucial Market," March 18, 2015, http://www.mhealthnews.com/news/smartwatches-are-missing-crucial-market, accessed November 22, 2015. See also Accenture, "Silver

Surfers Are Catching the e-Health Wave," http://www.accenture.com/us-en/Pages/insight-silver-surfer-catching-ehealth-wave.aspx, accessed March 20, 2015.

20. Elizabeth Wissinger, *This Year's Model: Fashion, Media, and the Making of Glamour* (New York: NYU Press, 2015), 275.

21. Carl Cederström and André Spicer, *The Wellness Syndrome* (London: Polity, 2015).

22. Steven Poole, "The Wellness Syndrome by Carl Cederström & André Spicer," *The Guardian*, January 22, 2015, http://www.theguardian.com/books/2015/jan/22/the-wellness-syndrome-carl-cederstrom-andre-spicer-persuasive-diagnosis/, accessed December 14, 2015.

23. Sarah O'Connor, "Wearables at Work: The New Frontier of Employee Surveillance," June 8, 2015, http://www.ft.com/intl/cms/s/2/d7eee768-0b65-11e5-994d-00144feabdc0.html, accessed December 13, 2015.

24. Simon Head, *Mindless: Why Smarter Machines are Making Dumber Humans* (New York: Basic Books, 2014), 3.

25. ABI Research, "Corporate Wellness Is a 13 Million Unit Wearable Wireless Device Opportunity," September 25, 2013, https://www.abiresearch.com/press/corporate-wellness-is-a-13-million-unit-wearable-w/, accessed December 14, 2015.

26. See Al Lewis and Vik Khanna, "Corporate Wellness Programs Lose Money," *Harvard Business Review*, October 15, 2015, https://hbr.org/2015/10/corporate-wellness-programs-lose-money?cm_sp=Article-_-Links-_-Top%20of%20Page%20Recirculation; and Leonard Berry, Ann Mirabito, and William Baun, "What's the Hard Return on Employee Wellness Programs, *Harvard Business Review*, December 2010, https://hbr.org/2010/12/whats-the-hard-return-on-employee-wellness-programs, both accessed December 14, 2015.

27. Scott Berinato, "Corporate Wellness Programs Make Us Unwell: An Interview with André Spicer," May 2015, https://hbr.org/2015/05/corporate-wellness-programs-make-us-unwell, accessed December 13, 2015. See also Mitesh S. Patel et al., "Premium-Based Financial Incentives Did Not Promote Workplace Weight Loss in a 2013–15 Study," *Health Affairs* 35 (2016): 71–79, doi: 10.1377/hlthaff.2015.0945.

5 Self-Tracking and Medicine

1. Susannah Fox and Maeve Duggan, "Tracking for Health" (Washington, DC: Pew Research Center Internet & American Life Project, 2013), January

28, 2013, http://www.pewinternet.org/2013/01/28/main-report-8, accessed November 22, 2015.

2. Ibid.

3. See "'We Are Not Waiting'—Diabetes Data Innovation Now!", n.d., http://www.healthline.com/health/diabetesmine/innovation/we-are-not-waiting, accessed November 22, 2015.

4. See Kate Linebaugh, "Citizen Hackers Tinker with Medical Devices," *Wall Street Journal*, September 26, 2014, http://www.wsj.com/articles/citizen-hackers-concoct-upgrades-for-medical-devices-1411762843, accessed November 22, 2015. See also http://www.nightscout.info, accessed November 22, 2015.

5. Nanette Byrnes, "Vinod Khosla Predicts a Better, Mobile Future for Medicine," *MIT Technology Review*, July 21, 2014, http://www.technologyreview.com/news/529056/more-phones-fewer-doctors/, accessed November 22, 2015.

6. See the archived version of Scanadu's homepage, June 1, 2016, https://web.archive.org/web/20150601171354/https://www.scanadu.com/scout, accessed November 22, 2015.

7. Nanette Byrnes, "Can Mobile Technologies and Big Data Improve Health?" *MIT Technology Review*, July 21, 2014, http://www.technologyreview.com/news/529011/can-technology-fix-medicine/, accessed November 22, 2015.

8. Technology Advice, 2014, "Wearable Technology & Preventative Health Care: Trends in Fitness Tracking among US Adults," http://research.technologyadvice.com/wearable-technology-study/, accessed August 10, 2015.

9. Withings Health Institute, n.d., "White Paper on Connected Health: The Case for Medicine 2.0," http://www.academia.edu/9447836/WHITE_PAPER_ON_CONNECTED_HEALTH, accessed November 22, 2015.

10. Fox and Duggan, "Tracking for Health."

11. Anthony L. Back and Gina Neff, "New Roles for Physicians in the Era of Connected Patients," Stanford Medicine X 2014, https://www.youtube.com/watch?v=5O04ojBkWIU, accessed February 14, 2015.

12. Trans-NIH Workshop to Explore the Ethical, Legal and Social Implications (ELSI) of Citizen Science, January 14–15, 2015, http://www.genome.gov/27559982, accessed January 24, 2015. The working group differentiates citizen science from the older and more established methods of community-based and participatory research.

13. Jennifer Couch, "Lay of the Land for Citizen Science at NIH," January 13–14, 2015. https://www.youtube.com/watch?v=Fi1v1vPO8wM, accessed February 19, 2015.

14. Elizabeth Yeampierre, "Building the Relationship: Citizen and Community Engagement," January 23, 2015, https://www.youtube.com/watch?v=kCF6dIDcx0k, accessed February 19, 2015.

15. "Research That Moves Us," n.d., http://c3nproject.org/researchers, accessed November 22, 2015.

16. Brittany Fiore-Gartland and Gina Neff, "Communication, Mediation, and the Expectations of Data: Data Valences across Health and Wellness Communities," *International Journal of Communication* 9 (2015): 1466–1484, http://ijoc.org/index.php/ijoc/article/view/2830, accessed November 22, 2015.

17. Michael E. Copeland, "New App Turns Your Phone into a Mobile Urine Lab," *Wired*, February 26, 2013, http://www.wired.com/2013/02/smartphone-becomes-smart-lab/, accessed January 9, 2016.

18. "UChek: A Mobile App to Test Urine," March 4, 2014, http://tedxtalks.ted.com/video/uChek-a-mobile-app-to-test-urin, accessed August 10, 2015.

19. Chris Pruitt, "Lessons from FDA's first Public Mobile Medical Apps Enforcement Letter," June 6, 2013, http://www.insidemedicaldevices.com/2013/06/06/lessons-from-fdas-first-public-mobile-medical-apps-enforcement-letter/, accessed August 10, 2015.

20. Dawn Lemanne, "A New Type of Evidence," Quantified Self Public Health Symposium, April 3, 2014, https://vimeo.com/130155293, accessed December 14, 2015.

21. Tara McCurdie, Svetlena Taneva, Mark Casselman, Melanie Yeung, Cassie McDaniel, Wayne Ho, and Joseph Cafazzo, "mHealth Consumer Apps: The Case for User-centered Design," *Biomedical Instrumentation and Technology* (Fall Supp. 2012): 49–56.

22. Fox and Duggan, "Tracking for Health," 11.

23. J. C. Herz, "Wearables Are Totally Failing the People Who Need Them Most," *Wired*, November 6, 2014, http://www.wired.com/2014/11/where-fitness-trackers-fail/, accessed November 22, 2015.

24. Anne Helen Peterson, "Big Mother Is Watching You: The Track-Everything Revolution Is Here Whether You Want It or Not," January 1, 2015, http://www.buzzfeed.com/annehelenpetersen/the-track-everything-revolution-is-here-to-improve-you-wheth#.mj20xaYQO, accessed January 24, 2015.

25. David F. Carr, "Quantified Self Should Be about Health, Not Ego," *InformationWeek*, September 25, 2014, http://www.informationweek.com/healthcare/patient-tools/quantified-self-should-be-about-health-not-ego-/a/d-id/1316069, accessed November 22, 2015.

26. Clinton Foundation 2015 Health Matters Activation Summit, https://www.youtube.com/watch?v=wTMyO61l0iE&feature=youtu.be, accessed February 23, 2015.

27. Parmy Olson and Aaron Tilley, "The Quantified Other: Nest and Fitbit Chase a Lucrative Side Business," *Forbes*, April 17, 2015, http://www.forbes.com/sites/parmyolson/2014/04/17/the-quantified-other-nest-and-fitbit-chase-a-lucrative-side-business/, accessed January 5, 2015.

28. Anni Ylagan and Andre Bierzynski, "Using Sensor Technology to Lower Elder Care Costs," July 28, 2014, http://deloitte.wsj.com/cio/2014/07/28/using-sensor-technology-to-lower-elder-care-costs/, accessed August 11, 2015.

29. Maggie Mort, Celia Roberts, and Blanca Callen, "Ageing with Telecare: Care or Coercion in Austerity?," *Sociology of Health & Illness* 35 (2013): 799–812.

6 Future Directions for Self-Tracking

1. Ernesto Ramirez and Hugo Campos, "My Device, My Body, My Data: An Access Conversation with Hugo Campos," February 4, 2015, https://medium.com/access-matters/my-device-my-body-my-data-4e158f8dfcec, accessed November 22, 2015.

2. "Hugo Campos Fights for the Right to Open His Heart's Data," January 20, 2012, http://tedxtalks.ted.com/video/TEDxCambridge-Hugo-Campos-fight, accessed November 22, 2015.

3. Mario Ballano Barcena, Candid Wueest, and Hon Lau, "How Safe Is Your Quantified Self?," *Security Response*, August 11, 2014, http://www.symantec.com/connect/blogs/how-safe-your-quantified-self-tracking-monitoring-and-wearable-tech, accessed December 17, 2015.

4. Edith Ramirez, "Privacy and the IoT: Navigating Policy Issues," Opening Remarks of FTC Chairwoman Edith Ramirez at the International Consumer Electronics Show, January 6, 2015, https://www.ftc.gov/public-statements/2015/01/privacy-iot-navigating-policy-issues-opening-remarks-ftc-chairwoman-edith, accessed December 17, 2015. See also Marguerite Reardon, "Tech Privacy Policies Need an Overhaul, Regulators Say," *CNet*, January 6, 2016, http://www.cnet.com/news/tech-privacy-policies-need-an-overhaul-regulators-say/, accessed January 16, 2016.

5. Gina Neff, "Why Big Data Won't Cure Us," *Big Data* (1): 117–123, doi:10.1089/big.2013.0029 2013.

6. The White House, "Big Data: Seizing Opportunities, Preserving Values," May 1, 2014, http://www.whitehouse.gov/sites/default/files/docs/big_data_privacy_report_5.1.14_final_print.pdf, accessed November 22, 2015. See also https://

www.eff.org/document/effs-comments-white-house-big-data, accessed March 29, 2015.

7. Dawn Nafus and Robin Barooah, "QSEU14 Breakout: Mapping Data Access," June 26, 2014, http://quantifiedself.com/2014/06/qseu14-breakout-mapping-data-access/, accessed December 14, 2015.

8. "Civil Rights Principles for the Era of Big Data," http://www.civilrights.org/press/2014/civil-rights-principles-big-data.html, accessed March 29, 2015.

9. The White House, "Big Data."

10. Ibid.

11. Kate Crawford and Jason Schultz, "Big Data and Due Process: Toward a Framework to Redress Predictive Privacy Harms," *Boston College Law Review* 55 (2014): 93–128.

12. See the work of Latayna Sweeney and the Data Privacy Lab at http://the datamap.org/risks.html, accessed November 22, 2015.

13. Myles Snyder, "Police: Woman's Fitness Watch Disproved Rape Report," June 19, 2015, http://abc27.com/2015/06/19/police-womans-fitness-watch-disproved-rape-report/, accessed November 22, 2015.

14. Kate Crawford, "When Fitbit Is the Expert Witness," *The Atlantic*, November 19, 2014, http://www.theatlantic.com/technology/archive/2014/11/when-fitbit-is-the-expert-witness/382936/, accessed February 27, 2015.

15. "FAA," http://vivametrica.com/grp_pages/faa/, accessed February 27, 2015.

16. Parmy Olson, "Fitbit Data Now Being Used in the Courtroom," *Forbes*, November 16, 2014, http://www.forbes.com/sites/parmyolson/2014/11/16/fitbit-data-court-room-personal-injury-claim/, accessed March 29, 2015.

17. Kim McAuliffe, "A Little Bit Pregnant," December 1, 2015, https://medium.com/@EnameledKoi/a-little-bit-pregnant-3122683ac793#.uvxss kozv, accessed December 14, 2015.

18. Wade Roush, "Linda Stone's Antidote to Quantified Self: The Essential Self," *Xconomy*, August 8, 2014, http://www.xconomy.com/national/2014/08/08/linda-stones-antidote-to-quantified-self-the-essential-self/, accessed February 25, 2015.

19. Dawn Nafus and Jamie Sherman, "This One Does Not Go Up to 11: The Quantified Self Movement as an Alternative Big Data Practice," *International Journal of Communication* 8 (2014): 1784–1794, http://ijoc.org/index.php/ijoc/article/view/2170, accessed November 22, 2015.

A/B testing   A form of experiment design intended to clarify the effects of a treatment or intervention, sometimes in a single person, by intentionally delineating between treatment periods and nontreatment periods. An A/B test looks for what happens before and after treatment, an A/B/A/B test adds another cycle of testing.

Accelerometer   A sensor commonly used in phones and wearable devices that tracks force and direction. Many different kinds of data are calculated from accelerometers, such as steps, activity levels, and orientation.

Activity tracker   A type of device for monitoring motion for people, usually connected to physical activity and exercise. Commercially available activity trackers include Jawbone's Up, the Fitbit, and Nike Fuelband. Several smart-watches and smartphones have activity-tracking capabilities built into them.

Aggregation   The process of bringing data together in some way. An aggregation could bring data together from many people. It could bring data together for one person, across many different sources. It could also be a way of processing data on an individual data stream, either by time (pulling out all the data that occurred between 5 pm and 6 pm), by place (all the data at home versus work), or value (all the data above a certain threshold).

Application Programming Interface (API)   A portal through which software developers can access a user's data and import it into their service. Depending on how an API is designed, handoffs between systems can occur at the request of the person who is the subject of the data or without her involvement.

Biomedicalization   The social process in which increasing areas of social life become dominated by medicalized and technological ways of understanding the world. Biomedicalization means both medicine and the technologies that are transforming medicine extend their jurisdiction beyond traditional problems of diseases and injury to more general notions of quality of life.

Citizen science   A situation where people without formal credentials take part in scientific research. Some citizen science projects contain participation by nonscientists in simple tasks like observation and data entry, while other projects involve nonprofessionals in research design, analysis, and dissemination.

Cloud   Industry term for the practice of storing data on server farms, as opposed to individual computers, phones, or smartwatches.

Compliance   The extent to which a patient follows medical prescription or advice.

Communal tracking   A method of citizen science that involves donating privately tracked data to public health research for the greater good.

Contextual integrity   An approach to understanding privacy that says privacy is maintained when data is kept in the social context in which it was produced, and where expectations and norms surrounding who has access to that data are upheld.

Datafication   The process by which data and data-driven decision making, as opposed to other kinds of knowing, become more important in society.

Enum   Data that contains a fixed repertoire of possible data points. An answer to a multiple-choice question would yield enum data. Often mood data is recorded in this way, from a fixed list of possible moods.

Exosense/exoself   Using available tools to create physically felt sensations that did not exist before.

Export   The ability to remove data from an application or service.

Gamification   The use of software interaction techniques derived from video games to persuade software users to perform a particular action.

Imposed tracking   When there is no meaningful alternative to tracking, such as when activity tracking becomes a prerequisite for employment or insurance coverage.

Interoperability According to the engineering standards body IEEE, interoperability is "the ability of two or more systems or components to exchange information and to use the information that has been exchanged."

Manual tracking Keeping track by writing something down or recording it in a spreadsheet or file, as opposed to tracking using digital sensors.

n **of 1** Personal experiments, where the number of subjects, or n, is only 1.

Pushed tracking Giving people incentives or social pressure to push people to track, such as when employers make it difficult for employees to choose not to track health or productivity.

Quantified Self The Quantified Self is a community of self-tracking enthusiasts founded by Gary Wolf and Kevin Kelly. The term "quantified self" (lowercase) is used by some journalists and academics to refer to self-tracking tools or related practices more broadly.

Sampling rate How often data is recorded or sampled by a sensor (e.g., every five minutes, every hour).

Sensor A small component of a device that detects some physical phenomena, like light, location or motion. A biosensor is a type of sensor that detects the presence of liquid or gas, like sweat or carbon dioxide.

Wearable A small computing device worn somewhere on the body; may refer to sensors and other devices worn as watches, jewelry, glasses, clothing, etc.

ADDITIONAL RESOURCES

On Self-Tracking in General

Dow-Schüll, Natasha. *Keeping Track: Personal Informatics, Self-Regulation, and the Data-Driven Life*. New York: Farrar, Straus, and Giroux, 2016.

Lupton, Deborah. *Quantified Self*. London: Polity, 2016.

Nafus, Dawn, ed. *Quantified: Biosensing Technologies in Everyday Life*. Cambridge, MA: MIT Press, 2016.

Self-Tracking and Health

Kay, Matthew, Dan Morris, and Julie A. Kientz. "There's No Such Thing as Gaining a Pound: Reconsidering the Bathroom Scale User Interface." In *Proceedings of the 2013 ACM International Joint Conference on Pervasive and Ubiquitous Computing*, 401–410. New York: ACM, 2013.

Neff, Gina. "Why Big Data Won't Cure Us." *Big Data* 1, no. 3 (2013): 117–123.

Robert Wood Johnson Foundation. "Personal Data for the Public Good: Final Report of the Health Data Project," March 2014. http://www.rwjf.org/en/library/research/2014/03/personal-data-for-the-public-good.html, accessed August 25, 2015.

Wolf, Gary, and Ernesto Ramirez. "Quantified Self Public Health Symposium Report," 2014. http://quantifiedself.com/symposium/Symposium-2014/QS PublicHealth2014_Report.pdf, accessed August 24, 2015.

Yom-Tov, Elad. *Crowdsourced Health: How What You Do on the Internet Will Improve Medicine* (Cambridge, MA: MIT Press, 2016).

Other Related Work

Hacking, Ian. *The Taming of Chance*. Cambridge: Cambridge University Press, 1990.

Joseph Dumit. "Illnesses You Have to Fight to Get: Facts as Forces in Uncertain, Emergent Illnesses." *Social Science & Medicine* 62 (2006): 577–590.

Clarke, Adele, J. Shim, L. Mamo, J. Fosket, and J. Fishman. *Biomedicalization: Technoscience and Transformations of Health and Illness in the US*. Durham, NC: Duke University Press, 2008.

Resources for Self-Tracking Projects

General

Duhigg, Charles. *The Power of Habit: Why We Do What We Do in Life and Business*. New York: Random House, 2012.

Examples of individual self-tracking projects, a library of self-tracking tools, and ongoing QS-related reading: http://quantifiedself.com/

Examples of n-of-1 experiments: http://blog.sethroberts.net/

How to do A/B experiment design: http://measuredme.com/2012/09/quantified -self-how-to-designing-self-experiment-html/

How to do case-crossover design: http://quantifiedself.com/2012/08/qs -primer-case-crossover-design/; http://www.pitt.edu/~super1/lecture/ lec0821/index.htm; http://quantifiedself.com/2012/08/qs-primer-case -crossover-design/

Data Coaching

Each of these resources has both a software interface to collect and view data, and a way of matching people with potential coaches.

Body Track Project, Carnegie Mellon University CREATE Lab, http://www .cmucreatelab.org/projects/BodyTrack

Coach.me: https://www.coach.me/

MyMee: http://www.mymee.com/whatwedo/

Data Crunching and Visualization

Data Sense: https://makesenseofdata.com/

Project Add App: https://addapp.io/

Tableau: http://www.tableau.com/

Zenobase: https://zenobase.com/

INDEX

Tag Heuer, 120
Technological solutionism, 111–112
Technology
  accelerometers and, 49, 60, 109
  apps and, 5, 11, 23, 28 (see also
    Apps)
  Bluetooth, 27, 109
  choice and, 41–42
  cloud computing and, 27
  consumers and, 105, 108,
    115–116, 121, 123, 125–126,
    128, 131–133
  continuous partial attention and,
    190
  data access and, 109, 113, 116,
    118, 120–125, 130
  data-driven innovation and,
    148–152
  developing countries and,
    184–185
  diabetes and, 121, 123, 133
  early abandonment and, 23–24
  electronics and, 18–19, 25, 27,
    137, 145, 156–157, 173
  experts and, 110, 118, 183
  fitness bands and, 2
  GPS and, 80, 109, 129
  healthcare system and, 108,
    121–124, 126, 140
  hype over, 6–7
  industry and, 23 (see also Indus-
    try)
  inflated sense of data's certainty
    and, 110–111, 119
  injury claims and, 182
  innovation and, 13, 34, 59, 105,
    109, 136, 139, 141, 148, 158,
    161, 183–184

  Internet and, 34, 113, 136–137,
    146, 173–174, 178–179
  lead users and, 21–23, 40
  machine vision software and,
    198n26
  makers/users boundary and, 109
  manufacturers and, 3, 41, 87, 110,
    121, 168, 173
  marketing and, 33, 105–106,
    116–119, 124–128, 141, 157,
    187
  maturation of, 109–110
  misuse of data and, 168–178, 182
  pattern analysis and, 116–119,
    123
  pedometers and, 31, 174
  privacy and, 105, 119, 132
  problem solving and, 111–112
  profit and, 61–63, 124–125, 136,
    157, 163, 184
  Quantified Self (QS) community
    and, 108–109, 190
  regulation and, 107, 123, 126,
    131–134
  security and, 105, 131–132
  sense of inadequacy and, 42
  sleep and, 126, 130
  smartphones and, 11, 14 (see also
    Smartphones)
  smart TVs and, 174
  smartwatches and, 2, 110, 120,
    138
  terms-of-service documents and,
    64–65, 117
  tinkering and, 69–70
  transducers and, 25, 155
  trough of disillusionment and, 6
  ubiquitous computing and, 27–28

GINA NEFF is Associate Professor of Communication and Sociology and a senior data scientist at the University of Washington. She is the author of *Venture Labor: Work and the Burden of Risk in Innovative Industries* (MIT Press). Dawn Nafus is Senior Research Scientist at Intel Labs and the editor of *Quantified: Biosensing Technologies in Everyday Life* (MIT Press).